EXERCISE
PHYSIOLOGY
STUDY GUIDE, WORKBOOK & LAB MANUAL

SIXTH EDITION

RANDY W. BRYNER ▸ DAVID A. DONLEY
West Virginia University School of Medicine

Kendall Hunt
publishing company

Cover images © Shutterstock, Inc.
All images are the authors unless otherwise noted.

Kendall Hunt
publishing company

www.kendallhunt.com
Send all inquiries to:
4050 Westmark Drive
Dubuque, IA 52004-1840

Copyright © 2009, 2011, 2012, 2013, 2015, 2018 by Kendall Hunt Publishing
Company

ISBN 978-1-5249-5861-9

All rights reserved. No part of this publication may be reproduced,
stored in a retrieval system, or transmitted, in any form or by any means,
electronic, mechanical, photocopying, recording, or otherwise,
without the prior written permission of the copyright owner.

Published in the United States of America

Contents

Preface V

How to Use This Text V

SECTION I

UNIT 1: ENERGY METABOLISM: PART I 1

Chapter 1:   Energy Value of Food 3

Chapter 2:   Introduction to Energy Transfer 7

Chapter 3:   Energy Transfer in the Body 13

UNIT 2: ENERGY METABOLISM: PART II 33

Chapter 4:   Energy Transfer in Exercise 35

Chapter 5:   Measurement of Energy Expenditure 49

Chapter 6:   Human Energy and Expenditure 57

UNIT 3: NEUROMUSCULAR PHYSIOLOGY AND EXERCISE 65

Chapter 7:   Skeletal Muscle 67

Chapter 8:   Neural Control of Human Movement 91

UNIT 4: CARDIOPULMONARY EXERCISE PHYSIOLOGY 105

Chapter 9:   General Overview of the Cardiovascular System 107

UNIT 5: CARDIOPULMONARY EXERCISE PHYSIOLOGY 145

Chapter 10:   Pulmonary Structure and Function 147

Chapter 11:   Gas Exchange and Transport 157

Chapter 12:   Pulmonary Ventilation 169

SECTION ONE: LABORATORY ASSIGNMENTS 177

Unit One Laboratories 177

Unit Two Laboratories 189

Unit Three Laboratories 203

Unit Four Laboratories 223

Unit Five Laboratories 231

iii

SECTION II

UNIT 1: EXERCISE AND THE ENDOCRINE SYSTEM.................. 237

Chapter 13: Exercise and the Endocrine System 239

UNIT 2: CLINICAL EXERCISE PHYSIOLOGY........................... 269

Chapter 14: Body Composition... 271

Chapter 15: Overweight, Obesity, and Weight Control 281

UNIT 3: EXERCISE PERFORMANCE AND ENVIRONMENTAL STRESS 311

Chapter 16: Exercise at Altitude.. 313

Chapter 17: Diving Depth and Pressure 317

Chapter 18: Microgravity.. 323

Chapter 19: Exercise and Thermal Stress.. 327

UNIT 4: EXERCISE IS MEDICINE... 345

Chapter 20: Electrocardiogram/Exercise for Rehabilitation 347

SECTION TWO: LABORATORY ASSIGNMENTS........................... 373

Unit One Laboratories 373

Unit Two Laboratories.. 389

Unit Three Laboratories.. 423

Unit Four Laboratories 429

Preface

Exercise Physiology Study Guide, Workbook and Lab Manual is a comprehensive book that provides material to be used in an Exercise Physiology course including a general overview of lecture notes, review questions that can be used to enhance student learning, and laboratory assignments which correspond to material being taught in class. The book is meant to be used as part of a two-semester course although it can be adapted for one semester courses. Critical concepts pertaining to the effects of exercise on physiological systems (Section/semester one) will serve as a foundation for the role of exercise as medicine for various disease populations (Section/semester two). The workbook contains daily outline notes that are to be used along with the professor's lectures. Although the outline notes are thorough they will require student participation to make them complete. In addition, another function of the workbook is to provide take home assignments that will assist in student learning, monitor student progress throughout the semester, and motivate regular attendance to class. Finally, the workbook contains laboratory assignments that are part of an Exercise Physiology curriculum and can be conducted in basic exercise physiology laboratories. The use of the study guide portion of the book with the weekly assigned laboratories will help broaden student's under-standing of the important concepts being presented during course lectures. Thorough use of this workbook will emphasize an active student learning environment which will help the student bridge the gap from basic concepts to integration and application of knowledge.

How to Use This Text

The purpose of this book is threefold. **First** it will serve as your daily note packet to be used in each class. Included in each *unit section*, you will find outline notes which corresponds with the professor's power point lectures, take home assignments, and unit extra credit crossword puzzles. You will need to use the outline notes each day during lectures. Assignments and extra credit will be periodically collected in class and used either for attendance purposes or as part of your overall grade. **Second**, this book will serve as a study guide for the course. Each section has highlighted *terms and concepts* to help focus your attention on important topics being discussed in class. In addition, review questions which include a variety of approaches to learning, such as multiple-choice, fill-in, matching, and short answer are included. Questions are derived from material found in lectures and other assigned readings given during class. **Third**, the book contains the labs that will be used in the laboratory section of the course. Students should bring the book with them each week and complete all assigned labs. These will be collected and graded and incorporated into the overall grade for this course.

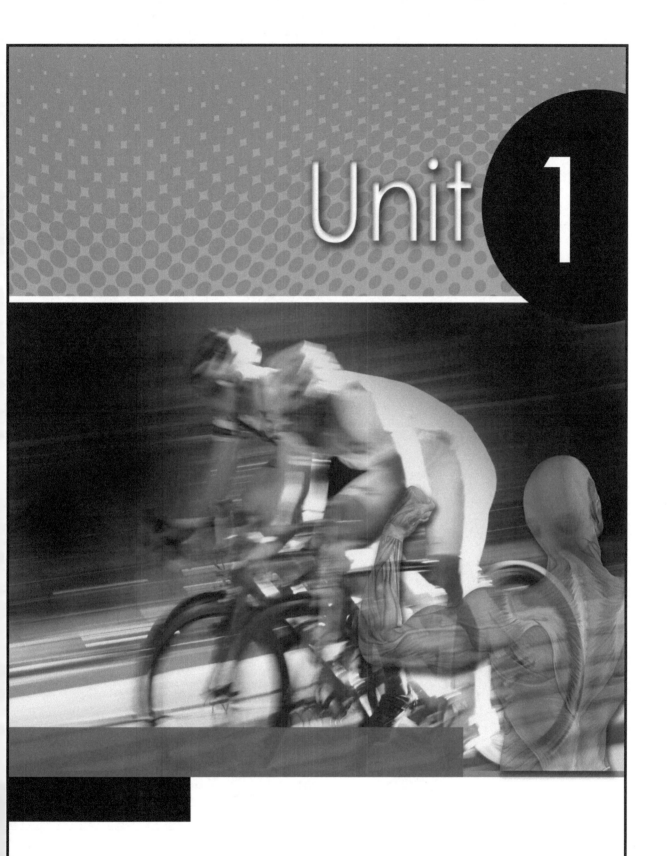

Unit 1

Energy Metabolism: Part I

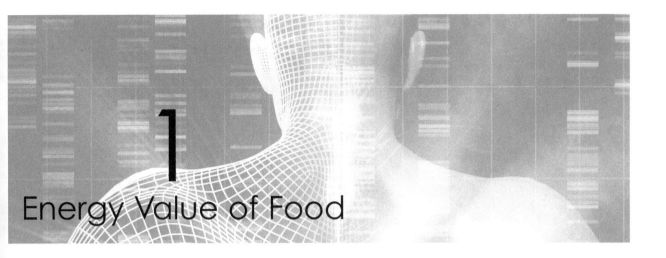

Energy Value of Food

The measurement of food energy is usually expressed in calories.

Kilocalorie:
- One calorie is the heat needed to raise the temperature of 1 kg (1 L) of water 1 °C. (specifically from 14.5 to 15.5 °C).
- Kilocalorie more accurately defines the calorific value of food.

A British thermal unit (BTU) is the quantity of heat required to raise the temperature of 1 pound of water by 1 °F from 63 to 64 °F.

Temperature: is a quantitative measure of an object's hotness or coldness

Heat: describes energy transfer or exchange from one body or system to another

Kilojoules: reflects the standard international unit to express food energy. (kcal × 4.184 = kJ)

- One J is the work done, or energy expanded, when one Newton of force acts through a distance of one meter: 1J = 1Nm.

The gross energy value of food is often determined in bomb calorimeters.

Bomb calorimeters operate on the principle of direct calorimetry which measures the heat liberated as food completely burns.

Heat of Combustion:
a. *Lipid*: varies with the structural composition of the fatty acid (average for 1 g fat is 9.4 kcal)

b. *Carbohydrate*: varies by structure (average for 1 g is 4.2 kcal)

c. *Protein*: depends on type of protein in food and relative nitrogen content (average for 1 g = 5.65 kcal)

(Lipids are more energy dense than carbohydrates or proteins because they have more hydrogen atoms that can be oxidized)

Net Energy Value of Foods:

Is the gross energy value of food (determined by heat of combustion) the same as the *net energy* available to the body?

- The heat of combustion value (gross energy value) determined by bomb calorimetry is not the same as the net energy value available to the body.

- This is especially true for protein because of the nitrogen content (approximately 19% loss of gross value)—4.6 kcal versus 5.65 kcal.

  - In the body, nitrogen atoms combine with hydrogen to form urea, which the kidneys excrete in the urine.

- The physiologic fuel values of CHO and fats are *identical* to their heats of combustion.

Coefficient of Digestibility:

The energy yield from food is in part determined by the efficiency of digestion.

Coefficient of Digestibility:

- Is the numeric value indicating the percentage of ingested food actually digested and absorbed to meet the body's metabolic need.

- The relative percentage of macronutrients digested and absorbed averages 97% for carbohydrate, 95% for lipid, and 92% for protein.

Atwater General Factors:

- Values which indicate the net metabolizable energy available to the body from ingested foods (CHO: 4 kcal/g; lipid: 9 kcal/g; protein: 4 kcal/g).

Review Questions for Chapter 1

1. One calorie is defined as the amount of heat required to raise ___ kg of water by ___ °C.

2. A. The sun transfers its energy to a car and subsequently warms it. The term that describes this process is:

   a. Temperature

   b. Heat

   B. This term describes how hot or cold an object is:

   a. Temperature

   b. Heat

3. The average heat of combustion for 1 g of lipid is approximately:

4. The average heat of combustion for 3 g of carbohydrate is approximately:

5. The average heat of combustion for 5 g of protein is approximately:

6. Explain the coefficient of digestibility.

7. Explain briefly why lipids contain more energy than carbohydrates or proteins.

8. On a particular food label you notice that for one serving there are 16 grams of carbohydrate, 9 grams of fat and 4 grams of protein. What is the total calories per serving?

2
Introduction to Energy Transfer

Bioenergetics:

All forms of biological work require power generated from the direct transfer of chemical energy.

Energy relates to a state of change, thus energy emerges only when a change occurs.

Energy relates to the ability to do work.

FIRST LAW OF THERMODYNAMICS:

Energy is neither created nor destroyed, but is transformed from one form to another (theory of conservation of energy).

Conservation of Energy:

Is illustrated when the body transforms energy in food to heat, mechanical, and chemical energy.

- Total energy of any system consists of two components:
    1. Potential energy: The energy that an object has due to its position in space (a skier at the top of a hill). It can also be relative to light, electric,or bound energy (a spring or a battery).
    2. Kinetic energy: The energy possessed by an object by virtue of its motion.

(* When potential energy is released, it is transformed into *kinetic energy or energy of motion.*)

Exergonic reactions—any physical or chemical process that results in the release (freeing) of energy to its surroundings.

$(\Delta G = \Delta H - T\Delta S)$

The ΔG will be negative during exergonic reactions because the product has less free energy than the reactant.

Chapter 2—Introduction to Energy Transfer   7

Endergonic reactions—chemical processes that store or absorb energy.

The ΔG will be positive during endergonic reactions because the product has more free energy than the reactant.

The capacity to do work always decreases during any spontaneous reactions that transfer potential energy.

SECOND LAW OF THERMODYNAMICS:

The tendency of potential energy to degrade to kinetic energy with a lower capacity to do work describes the second law of thermodynamics. (*Ultimately, all potential energy in a system degrades to the unusable form of kinetic or heat energy* i.e., increases entropy).

Interconversions of Energy:

- Photosynthesis

  - Captures energy that we utilize as food and oxygen

- Cellular respiration

  - Part of the energy released becomes conserved in compounds used for biologic processes

Factors That Affect the Rate of Bioenergetics:

- Enzymes: a highly specific and *large protein* catalyst, which accelerates the forward and reverse rates of chemical reactions within the body without being consumed or changed in the reaction (are not altered by the reaction they affect, therefore enzymes have a slow turnover rate and an enhanced ability to be reused).

- Enzymes lower the required **activation energy** and catalyze reactions 10^6 to 10^{20} faster than reactions which are uncatalyzed.

All enzymes do not operate at the same rate; some are slow while others operate quite quickly.

- Reaction rates depend upon:

  - pH

  - Temperature

  - Availability of substrates

Mode of Action:

- Lock and key mechanism (*active site*)

- Enzyme–substrate complex

  Coenzyme—nonprotein organic substances that facilitate enzyme action by binding the substrate with its specific enzyme.

  Oxidation reaction—reactions that transfer oxygen atoms, hydrogen atoms, or electrons. (A loss of electrons always occurs in oxidation reactions, with a corresponding gain in valence.)

Reduction reaction—involves any process in which the atoms in an element gain electrons, with a corresponding decrease in valence.

Reducing agent—describes the substance that donates or loses electrons as it oxidizes.

Oxidizing agent—is the substance being reduced or gaining electrons.

Redox reaction—oxidation and reduction reactions that occur together.

Reduction reaction:	Oxidation reaction:

Acid—any substance that ionizes in solution to give off H^+.

Base—any substance that forms hydroxide ions (OH^-) in a water solution.

Buffer—a chemical or physiological mechanism that prevents changes in the H^+ concentration and therefore pH.

Hydrolysis—a process by which complex organic molecules such as carbohydrates, lipids, and proteins are degraded or catabolized into simpler forms that the body can use with the use of water.

Thermodynamics:

1. All chemical reactions involve energy changes.

2. Chemical reactions in living organisms are catalyzed by enzymes.

3. Enzymes attempt to drive the reactions they catalyze toward equilibrium.

4. As enzyme-catalyzed reactions proceed toward equilibrium, they release energy.

5. The farther a reaction is from equilibrium, the more energy it can release.

6. Some energy released in a chemical reaction can be used to do useful work: the remainder is unavailable.

Chapter 2—Introduction to Energy Transfer   9

Review Questions for Chapter 2

(For true and false questions that are false, indicate what would make the question true)

1. Energy relates to the ability to do _____.

2. Define the first law of thermodynamics and give an example.

3. An object is dropped from the top of building. Once the object is released and is halfway from the ground, the object has (according to the conservation of energy):

   a. Potential energy only

   b. Kinetic energy only

   c. Potential energy and kinetic energy

4. When a lipid molecule is broken down, energy is subsequently released. This is an example of an _____.

   a. Exergonic reaction

   b. Endergonic reaction

5. *True or False*: The second law of thermodynamics states that the transfer of potential energy in any spontaneous process always proceeds in a direction that increases the capacity to perform work.

6. _____ and _____ are examples of energy conversion.

7. *True or False*: Enzymes are consumed during a reaction.

8. Briefly describe how enzymes increase the rate of the forward and reverse reactions.

9. Reaction rates depend on what three factors?

10. A. Pyruvate gains two hydrogens and thus forms lactate. This reaction is known as a _____ reaction.

    a. Oxidation

    b. Reduction

    B. In this example, pyruvate is being _____.

    a. Oxidized

    b. Reduced

11. What are the three types of biological work in humans? Give an example of each?

12. Briefly explain the purpose of a buffer.

Chapter 2—Introduction to Energy Transfer   11

Matching

13. Involves any process in which the atoms in an element gain electrons, with a corresponding decrease in valence.

    a. Oxidation reaction

14. Refers to the substance being reduced

    b. Reduction reaction

15. Any substance that ionizes in solution to give off H^+

    c. Reducing agent

16. Oxidation and reduction reactions that take place together

    d. Oxidizing agent

17. The term that refers to gain of electrons

    e. Redox reaction

18. Refers to the substance being oxidized

    f. Reduction

19. Reactions that transfer oxygen, hydrogen atoms or electrons. (A loss of electrons, with a corresponding gain in valency.)

    g. Oxidation

20. Any substance that forms hydroxide ions (OH^-) in a water solution

    h. Acid

21. The term that refers to the loss of electrons

    i. Base

22. What is the mechanism involved in hydrolysis and what is an example of hydrolysis?

    a. A water molecule forms as more complex molecules are formed; digestion

    b. A water molecule forms as more complex molecules are formed; forming nutrients

    c. The H^+ and OH^- from water are used to split chemical bonds; digestion

    d. The H^+ and OH^- from water are used to split chemical bonds; forming nutrients

23. *True or False*: The farther a reaction is from equilibrium, the more energy it can release.

24. *True or False*: Enzymes attempt to drive the reaction they catalyze toward equilibrium.

3
Energy Transfer in the Body

- Metabolism is the sum of all the chemical reactions that take place in a living organism.

- The human body must be continually supplied with chemical energy to perform activities.

- This chemical energy is generated by reactions inside and outside of cells.

What is the major difference between consuming glucose in a fire and within the skeletal muscle?

Where Does Energy Come From?

- Energy from food is not transported directly to cells for work. Chemical energy trapped within the carbohydrates, lipids, and proteins is extracted in relatively small quantities to power all biological reactions.

- The nutrient energy is stored in the energy-rich compound— **adenosine triphosphate** or ATP.

- The potential energy in ATP is used by all cells' energy requiring processes. ATP is formed from a molecule of adenine and ribose, called adenosine, which is linked to three phosphate molecules.

What are the outer two bonds in a molecule of ATP considered and why?

Draw an ATP Molecule:

- Through the process of hydrolysis and the aid of ATPase, energy is released from ATP.

Chapter 3—Energy Transfer in the Body   13

ATP Hydrolysis:

- ATP is therefore considered a ***high-energy phosphate compound***.

- **ATPase** is the enzyme that catalyzes this reaction.

- When ATP is hydrolyzed, **adenosine diphosphate** or **ADP** is formed and approximately 7.3 kcal of free energy is produced for every ATP molecule degraded to ADP.

- In intracellular environments, the actual free energy change has been determined to be 10 to 11 kcal/mole.

    - ATP + H_2O ⇔ ADP + P + Energy

- Notice there is *no oxygen* involved in the hydrolysis of ATP. This reaction **does not** require oxygen and is therefore said to be *anaerobic*, and the process is immediate.

- The energy released from ATP is harnessed by the body and used to power all forms of biological work within the body.

- Because energy is released from ATP, the reaction is said to be an **exergonic** reaction.

- The energy released from ATP can be used to power **endergonic** reactions.

    What is another name for exergonic reactions? Endergonic reactions?

- Because oxygen is not required for the breakdown of ATP, cells can liberate energy *immediately*.

- Therefore all types of exercise can be performed immediately without consuming oxygen for short periods of time.

Cellular Site of ATP Synthesis:

Cytosol:

Mitochondria:

Does the Cell Store a Lot of ATP?

- Only a small quantity of ATP is actually stored within the cell (approximately, 80 to 100 g). *Therefore, it must be continually synthesized.*

- However, the intramuscular values decrease very little even during exercise.

- A change in the ATP/ADP ratio is an important metabolic signal indicating enhanced cellular metabolism.

- A change in the ATP/ADP ratio stimulates the breakdown of other stored energy-containing compounds.

Creatine Phosphate (CP):

- Some energy for ATP synthesis is supplied directly and rapidly by the *anaerobic splitting* of a phosphate molecule from another energy-rich compound called **creatine phosphate.**

14   Chapter 3—Energy Transfer in the Body

- CP has a higher *free energy* of hydrolysis than ATP. There is also more CP stored in the body than ATP.

- Energy is released when creatine is split from the phosphate. This energy can be used to resynthesize ATP.

- Notice once again, the CP reaction *does not* require oxygen and is said to be an *anaerobic reaction*.

Adenylate Kinase Reaction:

Represents another single-enzyme-mediated reaction for ATP regeneration.

$$2ADP \Leftrightarrow ATP + AMP$$

Controlled by adenylate kinase.

- The energy released from the breakdown of the energy-rich phosphates, ATP and CP, can sustain all-out exercise, such as running, for approximately **8 to 10** seconds.

- If an all-out effort must be continued for more than 10 seconds, or if moderate exercise continues for much longer periods, an additional energy source is required to synthesize ATP.

- If this does not happen then the fuel supply will become depleted and movement will cease.

- Knowing the source of energy that a particular activity requires becomes very important.

   Why are the immediate energy sources so important to the muscle?

Phosphorylation: is the transfer of energy in the form of high-energy phosphate bonds (ATP and CP reactions).

- The energy for phosphorylation is ultimately generated by the oxidation ("biologic burning") of carbohydrates, lipids, and proteins.

Cellular Oxidation: is the crucial mechanism for energy metabolism in the body.

- Cellular oxidation–reduction constitutes the biochemical mechanism that underlies energy metabolism.

   What is the importance of the mitochondria?

- Hydrogen atoms are continually being stripped from carbohydrates, lipids, and proteins during energy metabolism. The process of removing H^+ and electrons begins in the cytoplasm.

- Carrier molecules within the mitochondria then remove electrons from these hydrogen atoms and pass them to molecular oxygen, which also accepts the H^+ atoms to form H_2O. Energy is released from this "electron transport system" to form ATP.

   Why is the transport of H^+ and electrons so important to the cell?

- *Dehydrogenase enzymes* catalyze the release of hydrogen atoms from nutrient substrates.

- The electrons from the hydrogen atoms are picked up in pairs by the coenzyme part of the dehydrogenase.

- **Nicotinamide adenine dinucleotide** or **NAD⁺**. NAD⁺ is gaining a hydrogen and two electrons and is being reduced to NADH. The other hydrogen appears in ionized form in the cell fluid as H⁺.
- **Flavin adenine dinucleotide** or **FAD**.

Unlike NAD⁺, FAD accepts both hydrogens to become $FADH_2$.

- Each of these coenzymes becomes energy-rich molecules because they carry electrons that have high-energy transfer potential.
- Pairs of electrons carried by NADH and $FADH_2$ are passed to *cytochromes* (iron–protein electron carriers) on the inner mitochondrial membrane.

Respiratory Chain:

- The transport of electrons from hydrogen to oxygen by specific carrier molecules (cytochromes).
- For each pair of hydrogen atoms, two electrons flow down the chain and reduce one atom of oxygen to form H_2O.
- Free energy is released during this process.

Oxidative Phosphorylation:

- Oxidative phosphorylation is the process by which ATP is synthesized during the transfer of electrons from NADH and $FADH_2$ to molecular O_2.
- This process is separate from electron transport, but dependent on electron transport.
- The electron transport causes a proton gradient across the inner mitochondrial membrane, which results in a net flow of protons that provides the coupling mechanism to drive ATP synthesis.
- For every NADH and H⁺ in the electron transport chain, you get **three ATPs** produced.
- For every FADH in the electron transport chain, you get **two ATPs** produced.
- The final electron acceptor in the electron transport chain is oxygen and ultimately water is produced.

There are three conditions that must be met for oxidative phosphorylation to occur:

- A reducing agent in the form of NADH or $FADH_2$ must be available.
- An oxidizing agent (oxygen) must be present in the tissues.
- Enzymes must be present in sufficient concentrations to make the energy transfer reactions go forward.
- Oxygen functions to accept electrons (final electron acceptor) and forms H_2O.
- **Aerobic metabolism:** The process of coupled oxidative phosphorylation with oxygen serving as the final electron and H⁺ acceptor.

Why is oxidative phosphorylation so important to the cell?

Energy Release From Food:

- The energy release from the breakdown of food nutrients serves one purpose, to phosphorylate ADP and form ATP.

Carbohydrates:

- Primary function is to supply energy for cellular work.

- Is the only nutrient whose stored energy can be used to generate ATP **anaerobically** (important during heavy or intense exercise).

- During light to moderate exercise, carbohydrates supply about one-third of the body's energy needs.

- A continual breakdown of some CHO must occur so that fat nutrients can be used for energy.

- With the breakdown of each glucose molecule in the muscle cell, 263 kcal of energy are gained; therefore 36 moles of ATP are generated (263/7.3 = 36). (263 kcal/686 kcal = 38%)

- There are two stages for glucose degradation in the body: **anaerobic (fast) and aerobic (slow).**

Anaerobic:

- *Glycolysis:* When a glucose molecule enters a cell to be used for energy it undergoes a series of chemical reactions.

- *Glycogenolysis:* When the series of reactions starts with stored glycogen. This is the breakdown of glycogen into glucose for energy.

- Glycogen breakdown is regulated by **phosphorylase**. The activity of this enzyme is greatly influenced by **epinephrine** (activity goes up during physical activity/exercise).

  - Release of Ca^+ and phosphate ions is also important.

- Glycogen formation is under the influence of **glycogen synthase** (activity goes up following a meal).

Glycolysis:

- Glycolysis is a series of controlled chemical reactions that occur during the anaerobic breakdown of glucose, which occurs in the cytoplasm of the cell.

- In Step 1, ATP is required to break down glucose into glucose 6-phosphate. Because energy must be added, this step is endergonic.

- In Step 3, ATP is once again required for the breakdown of fructose 6-phosphate to fructose 1,6-diphosphate. This step requires the enzyme **phosphofructokinase**, which may place a limit on glycolysis during all-out exercise.

- In Step 5, fructose 1,6-diphosphate, which is a 6-carbon molecule, is being broken down into two 3-carbon molecules. Now there are *two* 3-phosphoglyceraldehyde molecules.

Chapter 3—Energy Transfer in the Body   17

- In Steps 7 and 10, two molecules of ATP are being produced in each step, for a total of four ATPs produced by the process of anaerobic glycolysis.

- However, do not forget that Steps 1 and 3 required the addition of ATP.

- Therefore, the **net gain** of ATP molecules during anaerobic glycolysis is **two**. Four ATP produced but two lost in Steps 1 and 3 for a net total of two ATP by the anaerobic process of substrate phosphorylation. **(Energy conservation during glycolysis operates at an efficiency of approximately 30%.)**

Draw and label the important steps of glycolysis:

- This process accounts for only approximately **5%** of the total ATP generated in the complete breakdown of a glucose molecule.

- This process is a very rapid series of reactions and is therefore utilized during exercise of high intensity (e.g., extra kick at the end of a mile, or a 40-yard sprint).

Why is a constant supply of carbohydrate to the skeletal muscle so important?

Hydrogen Release During Glycolysis:

- Notice that two pairs of H^+ atoms are released and electrons passed to NAD^+ in Step 6 of glycolysis.

- Remember, normally if these electrons go to the respiratory chain, three molecules of ATP are formed from each molecule of NADH oxidized.

- However, the mitochondria are impermeable to the NADH formed in the cytoplasm during glycolysis. Therefore, the electrons from the NADH produced during glycolysis must be shuttled indirectly into the mitochondria.

- In skeletal muscle, this is accomplished by the **glycerol phosphate** shuttle. This shuttle transfers a less reduced version of NADH. Therefore, only two ATPs, rather than three, are formed when cytosolic NADH is oxidized by the respiratory chain. (malate–aspartate shuttle predominates in the heart, kidney, and liver cells.)

- Therefore, *a total of four ATP* molecules are formed aerobically from glycolysis because two molecules of NADH ($FADH_2$) are formed during anaerobic glycolysis.

Draw the two shuttle system:

Lactic Acid:

- When plenty of oxygen is available or glycolysis is slowed, most of the hydrogens (electrons) stripped from glucose are carried by NADH and oxidized within the mitochondria and passed to oxygen to form water. This is often referred to as **aerobic glycolysis**.

- However, during strenuous exercise, when energy demands exceed either the oxygen supply or *its rate of utilization*, the rate of production of hydrogen joined to NADH exceeds the rate at which it can be processed through the respiratory chain.

- This back up of NADH combines with the end product of glycolysis, pyruvic acid, and forms lactic acid.

How did Lucy inadvertently create lactic acid?

What is the chemical formula for lactic acid?

- Even at rest and during light exercise, lactic acid is **always** being produced. However, during these times in which oxygen is not limited, any lactic acid that is produced is oxidized by tissues at its rate of formation. Therefore, its production rate is equal to its removal rate.

- When NADH + H^+ combines with pyruvic acid to form lactic acid this is known as *anaerobic glycolysis*.

Chapter 3—Energy Transfer in the Body   19

- Lactic acid rapidly diffuses into the blood thereby increasing the pH of the blood because lactic acid is buffered within the blood to form **lactate**. The increased lactate concentration causes an *increase* in blood pH.

- However, when lactic acid production exceeds the rate at which it is being buffered, the blood becomes more acidic.

- Increased acidity is believed to be partially responsible for fatigue during exercise because it can inactivate various enzymes involved in energy transfer.

- Is lactic acid a metabolic waste product? Why?

- When sufficient O_2 is once again present, during recovery, the H^+ atoms from lactic acid are picked up by the NAD^+ and oxidized.

- Lactic acid and pyruvate can be converted to glucose (gluconeogenesis) by a process known as the **Cori cycle** within the liver.

- The Cori cycle is a biochemical process in which the lactic acid released from active tissues is taken to the **liver** via the bloodstream and converted to glucose.

- Important for replenishing glycogen levels which might have become depleted during long exercise.

- This glucose may also be used for immediate energy by going through the process of glycolysis.

Summary of Lactic Acid:

KREBS CYCLE (Citric Acid or Tricarboxylic Acid Cycle):

- Only approximately 5% of the energy within a glucose molecule is released during anaerobic glycolysis.

- When sufficient oxygen is present, the pyruvic acid formed during the glycolysis of a glucose molecule is converted to acetyl-CoA. This molecule then enters the **Krebs cycle**.

- The main function of the Krebs cycle is to degrade the acetyl-CoA to CO_2 and H atoms within the mitochondria.

- Pyruvic acid joins with vitamin B derivative coenzyme A and forms acetyl-CoA.

- For each molecule of acetyl-CoA oxidized in the Krebs cycle, two CO_2 molecules and four pairs of hydrogen atoms are cleaved from the substrate

- The H atoms that are cleaved from the substrate combine with NAD^+ and FAD to be carried to the respiratory chain.

- Notice that oxygen does not participate directly in the reactions of the Krebs cycle. However, most of the energy generated from pyruvate is generated in the aerobic process of electron transport and oxidative phosphorylation.

- Therefore, oxygen must be present for the Krebs cycle to proceed unimpeded.

Review of important steps in the Krebs cycle:

The citric acid cycle, electron transport system, and oxidative phosphorylation represent the three components of aerobic metabolism.

Total ATP produced from one molecule of glucose.

Substrate phosphorylation in glycolysis	2 ATP
2 NADH formed in glycolysis	4 ATP
2 NADH from pyruvate to acetyl-CoA	6 ATP
Substrate phosphorylation in Krebs	2 ATP
6 NADH and 2 FADH2 in Krebs	22 ATP
Total	36 ATP

Does exercise intensity affect muscle glucose use?

How does carbohydrate in the diet affect exercise performance?

Energy Release from Fat:

- The fat stored within the body's various compartments serves as the most plentiful source of potential energy.

  - In an adult male, average fuel reserve from fat is approximately 60,000 to 100,000 kcal (about 3,000 kcal from intramuscular triacylglycerol).

- The fuel reserve from CHO is about 2% of this, or approximately 2,000 kcal.

Sources of Lipid Catabolism or Breakdown:

- Triglycerides stored directly within the muscle cell, particularly the high oxidative (slow twitch) fibers.

- Circulating triglycerides in lipoprotein complexes, which are hydrolyzed by lipoprotein lipase on the surface of a tissue's capillary endothelium.

- Free fatty acids (FFA) mobilized from triglycerides in adipose tissue which circulate throughout the blood stream.

- The primary storage site of fatty acid molecules is **adipose tissue**.

Chapter 3—Energy Transfer in the Body   21

- Approximately 95% of an adipocyte, or fat cell, is stored triglyceride molecules.

- For energy release to occur from fat, the triglyceride molecule must be hydrolyzed in the cell's cytosol into glycerol and FFA molecules.

- Hormone-sensitive lipase (activated by cyclic AMP) catalyzes triacylglycerol breakdown as follows:

  - Once a triglyceride molecule is broken down into three fatty acids, the fatty acids leave the adipocyte and enter the blood stream.

  - Once in the blood stream, the fatty acids bind with albumin and become **FFA**. FFA in the circulation can be used for energy.

  - The use of FFA by tissues for energy varies closely with the amount of blood flow. As blood flow increases, more FFAs are delivered to the active muscles for energy.

  - This is especially important for **slow-twitch** muscle fibers because they have ample **blood supply** and **large, numerous mitochondria** which make them ideal for the purpose of lipid catabolism.

  - Depending on an individual's state of nutrition and fitness and the level and duration of physical activity, 30 to 80% of the energy for biological work can be derived from fat sources.

  - Fat becomes the primary energy fuel for exercise and recovery when high-intensity, long-duration exercise depletes glycogen.

  - *Epinephrine, norepinephrine, glucagon*, and *growth hormone* all activate the enzyme **lipase**, which converts triglycerides to glycerol and fatty acids.

Catabolism of Glycerol and Fatty Acids:

Glycerol:

- Glycerol can be accepted into the anaerobic reaction of glycolysis as 3-phosphoglyceraldehyde and converted to pyruvic acid (Step 6 in glycolysis).

- How many ATP molecules would this provide?

- Remember, there is only one molecule of 3-phosphoglyceraldehyde entering glycolysis and therefore only one molecule of pyruvic acid is going to be formed.

- Glycerol can also provide its carbon skeleton for glucose synthesis.

- This is important when carbohydrates are restricted in the diet or during long-term exercise, which might drain glycogen stores.

- Would taking glycerol as an energy supplement during exercise enhance performance?

Beta Oxidation:

- Beta oxidation is the breakdown of a fatty acid molecule within the mitochondria. A fatty acid molecule is composed of a long carbon chain.

- In beta oxidation, the fatty acid molecule is successively cleaved into two carbon acetyl fragments to form acetyl-CoA.

- This acetyl-CoA is the same molecule that enters the Krebs cycle.

Must have oxygen present for beta oxidation to occur in order to accept the hydrogens.

Draw the Basic Components of Lipolysis:

What is the total ATP yield for a **triglyceride** molecule which contains three 18-carbon fatty acids?

For an 18-carbon fatty acid:

18 carbons—9 acetyl units	
Cycles through beta oxidation—8 cycles	
Each 8 cycles → 1 $FADH_2$ (8 × 2)	16 ATP
Each 8 cycles → 1 NADH (8 × 3)	24 ATP
Each of 9 Acetyl-CoA entering Krebs cycle → 12ATP/ acetyl-CoA (12 × 9)	108 ATP
16 + 24 + 108 = 148 ATP − 1ATP for activation	147 ATP
Because there are three fatty acid molecules for each triglyceride molecule (147 × 3)	441 ATP
441 ATP + 19 ATP from glycerol catabolism,	**460 ATP**

Chapter 3—Energy Transfer in the Body   23

How does exercise duration and intensity influence free fatty use? Does training have an effect?

Factors Associated with Enhanced FFA Use:

1. Enhanced rate of lipolysis within adipose tissue.
2. Increased capillary density within the muscle.
3. Improved transport of FFA through the muscle fiber membrane.
4. Increased carnitine and carnitine acyltransferase.
5. Increased size and number of mitochondria.
6. Increased quantity of mitochondrial enzymes.

Energy Release from Proteins:

- Protein can serve an important role as an energy substrate during substantial exercise and heavy training (primarily the branched-chain amino acids, leucine, isoleucine, valine, glutamine, and aspartate).
- Nitrogen must be removed (*deamination*) so amino acid can enter pathways for energy release.
- The main site for *deamination* is the liver.
- Muscles also contain enzymes for the removal of nitrogen.
- This process is called *transamination*.
- Some amino acids are *glucogenic*, which means they provide the intermediates for glucose synthesis.
- Does nutrition affect protein use during exercise?

The Metabolic Mill:

- Describes how CHO, fats, and proteins are interchangeably used for energy.
- Fat burns in a carbohydrate flame.
- This is because fatty acid breakdown depends in part on a continual level of carbohydrate catabolism.
- The degradation of fatty acids via the Krebs cycle continues only if sufficient oxaloacetate is available to combine with the acetyl-CoA from beta oxidation.
- Acetyl-CoA enters the Krebs cycle by combining with oxaloacetate to form citrate.
- This oxaloacetate is generated from pyruvate during carbohydrate (glucose) breakdown under the control of the enzyme pyruvate carboxylase.
- Therefore, fat burns in a carbohydrate flame.

24   Chapter 3—Energy Transfer in the Body

Which fuel would be used primarily during the following situations?

a. 400-m sprint

b. 60-m sprint

c. 5-mile run

What controls metabolism?

- By far, the most important factor that controls the breakdown of carbohydrates, fat, and amino acids for energy release in the cell is the concentration of cellular ADP.

- Other important factors include the NADH/NAD ratio, intracellular calcium, citrate, and pH.

- ATP and NADH inhibit enzymes.

- ADP, NAD, and intracellular calcium activate enzymes.

Recommended CHO Intake:

- For a 70-kg man:

    - 300 g or between 40 and 50% of total caloric intake.

- For physically active individuals:

    - 400 to 600 g or approximately 60% of daily calories (as unrefined, fiber-rich, grains, and vegetables).

- During periods of intense training:

    - 70% of total calories (8 to 10 g per kg of body mass)

Recommended Protein Intake:

- *Muscle mass does not increase simply by eating high-protein foods.*

- The RDA: 0.83 g of protein per kg body mass (i.e., 75 g for a 90-kg man).

- For individuals who train intensely, protein intake of 1.2 to 1.8 g of protein of body mass daily.

Low-Fat Diets:

- Restricting dietary fat below recommended levels (below 20%) can impair exercise performance.

CHO Feeding:

- One hour of intense aerobic exercise decreases liver glycogen by approximately 55%; 2 hours nearly depletes all of liver and active muscle glycogen.

- Consume a *low-glycemic* carbohydrate in the immediate 45 to 60-min **pre-exercise** period (want to prevent a rapid rise in insulin).

- Consume about 60 g of liquid or solid CHO each hour during high-intensity, long-duration aerobic exercise.

    - 5 to 8% CHO-electrolyte beverage

Chapter 3—Energy Transfer in the Body   25

- Consume a CHO-rich, *high-glycemic* food immediately **following** intense training to replenish glycogen.

Glycemic Index (GI):

- *Low GI*: beans, small seeds, most whole grains, most vegetables, most sweet fruits

- *High GI*: white bread, most white rice, corn flakes, glucose, maltose, potato, pretzels, bagels

Review Question for Chapter 3

(For true and false questions that are false, indicate what would make the question true)

1. What part of an ATP molecule contains stored energy?

2. A person ingests some food which is subsequently broken down to water and carbon dioxide. What is this process called? What type of reaction is this? What molecule does this result in?

   a. catabolism,   endergonic,   ADP + Pi

   b. anabolism,   endergonic,   ATP

   c. catabolism,   exergonic,   ADP + Pi

   d. catabolism,   exergonic,   ATP

   e. anabolism,   endergonic,   ADP + Pi

3. *True or False*: ATP break down is an aerobic process.

4. An athlete is sprinting for 8 to 10 seconds. His skeletal muscle cells contain a very small amount of ATP. When the initial supply of ATP is catabolized, a molecule is split to resynthesize ATP. What is the name of the molecule and the enzyme used in the reaction?

5. Does the athlete in question number 4 require oxygen? Why not?

6. When the myocardial tissue of the heart contracts, it allows blood to circulate throughout the body. What high-energy molecule is needed in order for this contraction to occur?

7. What reaction is occurring in the process of ATP synthesis via the enzyme creatine kinase?

8. In what organelle does the process of cellular oxidation take place?

   a. Endoplasmic reticulum

   b. Mitochondria

   c. Golgi apparatus

   d. Across the cell membrane

9. How much energy is released when the enzyme _____ splits ATP into _____ and Pi in vitro? in vivo?

10. Hydrogen atoms are stripped from carbohydrates, lipids, and proteins during energy metabolism. What type of enzyme catalyzes this reaction?

11. In the following reaction, NAD^+ is gaining a hydrogen and _____ electrons and is thus is being:

    a. Reduced

    b. Oxidized

    $$NAD^+ + H2 \longrightarrow NADH + H^+$$

Chapter 3—Energy Transfer in the Body   27

12. Briefly describe the *purpose* of the molecules NAD^+ and FAD^+. This process eventually leads to the production of what important molecule needed in almost all biological activity?

13. Briefly describe the mechanism that occurs in oxidative phosphorlyation, which enables ATP synthesis.

14. For every NADH and H^+ in the electron transport chain, _____ molecule(s) are produced

    a. 1 ATP

    b. 2 ATP

    c. 3 ATP

    d. 4 ATP

15. For every FADH in the electron transport chain, _____ molecule(s) are produced

    a. 1 ATP

    b. 2 ATP

    c. 3 ATP

    d. 4 ATP

16. a. What is the final electron acceptor in the electron transport chain? _____

    b. What are the final end-products of aerobic metabolism? _____.

17. What nutrient(s) stored energy can be used to generate ATP anaerobically?

    a. Carbohydrates

    b. Proteins

    c. Lipids

    d. a and c

    e. None of the above

18. Due to the excitement of competition, an athlete's sympathetic nervous system is stimulated. This causes an increase in circulating epinephrine. What metabolic changes will occur?

    a. Epinephrine will cause an increase in the activity of the enzyme phosphorylase, leading to glycogen synthesis.

    b. Epinephrine will cause an increase in the activity of the enzyme phosphorylase, leading to glycogen breakdown.

    c. Epinephrine will cause a decrease in the activity of the enzyme phosphorylase, leading to glycogen synthesis.

    d. Epinephrine will cause a decrease in the activity of the enzyme phosphorylase, leading to glycogen breakdown.

    e. No change will occur in glycogen synthesis.

19. Where does glycolysis occur?

    a. Outer mitochondrial membrane

    b. Cell wall

    c. Inner mitochondrial membrane

    d. Cytoplasm

20. During anaerobic glycolysis, the net gain in ATP molecules is ____

    a. 1

    b. 2

    c. 4

    d. 36

21. Oxidative phosphorylation produces about _____ % of total ATP generated while anaerobic glycolysis produces about ____ % of total ATP generated.

    a. 5%, 90%

    b. 90%, 5%

    c. 75%, 25%

    d. 25%, 75%

    e. None of the above

22. Briefly explain why lactic acid builds up during strenuous exercise.

23. *True or False*: Under normal conditions, lactic acid is always being produced.

24. *True or False*: Lactic acid is used by the liver as gluconeogenic precursor.

25. What molecule enters the Krebs cycle?

    a. Pyruvic acid

    b. Acetyl-CoA

    c. Glucose

    d. Pyruvate

    e. NAD^+ and FAD^+

26. *True or False*: Oxygen is not required for the Krebs cycle to proceed unimpeded.

Chapter 3—Energy Transfer in the Body   29

27. How many total molecules of NADH and $FADH_2$ are formed in the Krebs cycle?

    a. 6 NADH and 3 $FADH_2$

    b. 2 NADH and 6 $FADH_2$

    c. 3 NADH and 2 $FADH_2$

    d. 3 NADH and 3 $FADH_2$

    e. 6 NADH and 2 $FADH_2$

28. What two factors enable slow twitch muscle fibers to be ideal for lipid catabolism?

29. *True or False*: Fatty acid breakdown does not depend on carbohydrate catabolism.

30. What is the *most* important factor which determines the breakdown of carbohydrates, lipids, and amino acids for energy release?

    a. NADH/NAD ratio

    b. pH

    c. Cellular concentration of ADP

    d. Citrate

    e. Intracellular calcium

31. Why is the total ATP produced from a skeletal muscle cell different from a cardiac muscle cell?

32. What is the total ATP yield from a triglyceride whose fatty acid molecules are 22 carbon in length?

Unit 1

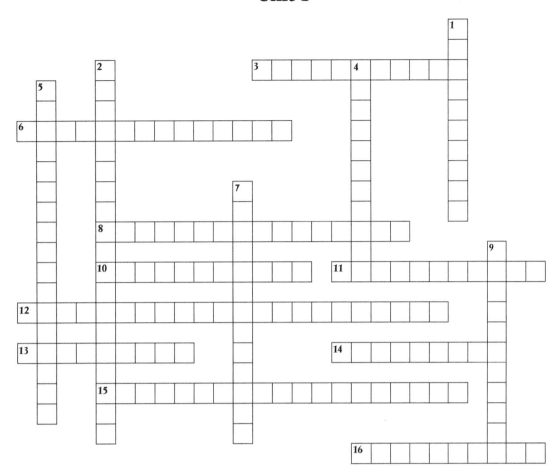

ACROSS

3 A sympathetic nervous system hormone.
6 The process of nitrogen removal from an amino acid and passing it to other compounds.
8 The final common pathway where electrons extracted from hydrogen pass to oxygen.
10 A series of iron-protein electron carriers dispersed on the inner membranes of the mitochondrion.
11 The process of nitrogen removal.
12 Stimulates fatty acids to diffuse from the adipocyte into circulation.
13 An intracellular mediator that activates hormone sensitive lipase and regulates fat breakdown.
14 The process that either oxidizes or synthesizes glucose from the latctate produced during exercise.
15 Lactate is the end product of this process.
16 The first stage of glucose degradation in a series of fermentation reactions.

DOWN

1 Second stage of carbohydrate breakdown, also called the Citric Acid Cycle.
2 Enzyme that controls the addition of a phosphate to a fructose 6-phosphate molecule forming fructose 1, 6-diphosphate.
4 Enzyme that splits the phosphate from glucose 6-phosphate.
5 Pyruvate is the end product of this process.
7 The process when a fatty acid molecule transforms to acetyl-CoA in the mitochondrion.
9 The formation of fat.

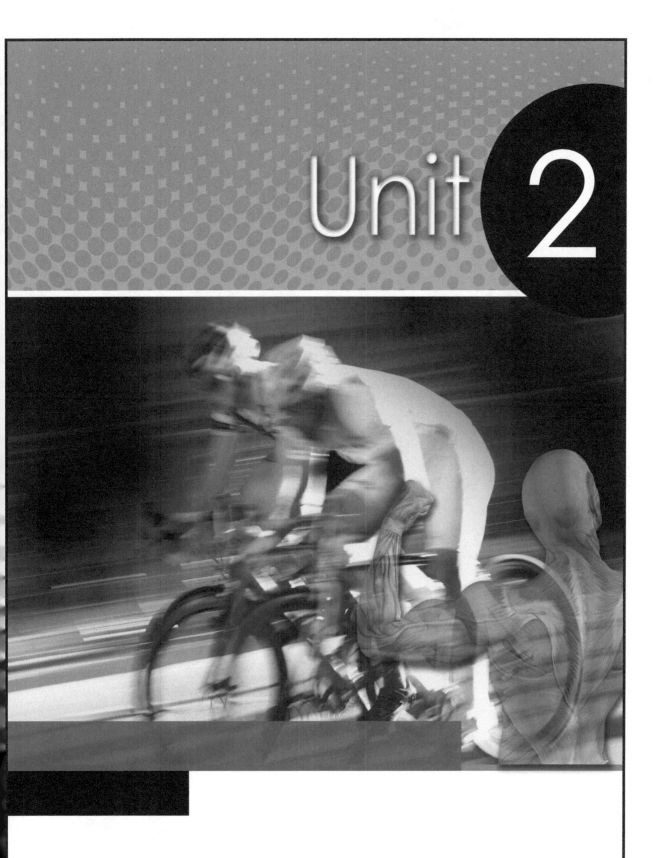

Unit 2

Energy Metabolism: Part II

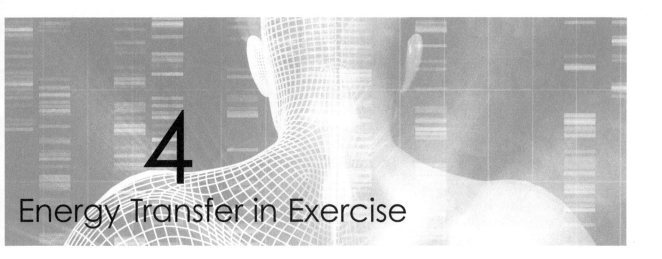

Energy Transfer in Exercise

The contributions from the various pathways of energy metabolism are dependent upon the intensity and duration of the exercise and the fitness level of the individual.

The ATP-CP System

- There is a very limited amount of high-energy phosphate (ATP and CP) stored within the muscle.
    - Approximately 3–8 mmol of ATP per kg of muscle (four to five times more PCr).
    - Enough to walk briskly for 1 minute, run a cross-country race for 20–30 seconds, or perform all-out exercise (sprint) for approximately 5–8 seconds.
    - The maximum rate of energy transfer from the intramuscular high-energy phosphates exceeds by 4 to 8 times the maximal energy transfer from aerobic metabolism.
    - In order to sustain exercise or recover from short all-out efforts, we must have a secondary energy source to replenish the ATP.
    - The energy to replace these high-energy phosphates during strenuous exercise comes primarily from glucose and stored glycogen during the anaerobic process of glycolysis, resulting primarily in the formation of lactic acid.

- The most rapidly accumulated and highest lactic acid levels are reached during **maximal exercise** that can be sustained for 60 to 180 seconds.

    What are the metabolic fates of lactic acid?

    Does lactic acid appear in the blood during all types of exercise?

    What are some of the causes of a greater lactic acid production during exercise?

- Blood lactate accumulates and rises in an exponential fashion at about 50–55% of the healthy, untrained person's maximal aerobic capacity.

- For a trained individual, the threshold for lactate buildup (termed either anaerobic threshold or blood lactate threshold) occurs at a higher percentage of the athlete's aerobic capacity.

- Possibly this is due to:

- Adaptations and increased removal may be caused by:

- These adaptations serve to increase the cells' capacity to generate ATP aerobically and delay the onset of blood lactate accumulation.

- Trained athletes can often perform at 80–90% of maximal capacity for aerobic metabolism before significant increases in blood lactate occur.

- Also, it is believed that training might enhance the ability to utilize lactic acid formed in one part of a working muscle by other fibers in the same muscle or other less active tissues (or by the muscle fiber itself).

- This is an important means of glucose conservation.

Lactate-Producing Capacity:

- After well-trained athletes perform maximal short-term exercise, their blood lactate levels are 20–30% higher than those of untrained subjects.

- Possibly due to:

Oxygen Consumption During Exercise:

- Steady State (Rate): Balance between the energy required by working muscles and the rate of ATP production via aerobic metabolism.

- Oxygen Deficit: "The difference between the total O_2 consumed during exercise and the total that would have been consumed had a steady rate of aerobic metabolism been reached immediately."

- Immediate energy for muscular work is always provided directly by the immediate and non-oxygen-consuming breakdown of ATP in muscle.

- The energy for the early stages of exercise (during the deficit) represents nonaerobic energy (stored phosphates and anaerobic glycolysis).

- Trained individuals will reach a steady state of O_2 consumption more rapidly than untrained individuals (e.g., smaller O_2 deficit).

Metabolic Composition of Muscle Skeletal Muscle Fibers:

- Fast-twitch (Type II)

  - Two basic subdivisions (IIa, IIx or IIb)

  - Possess a high capability for anaerobic production of ATP during glycolysis

    - Activated during change-of-pace (stop-and-go) activities (basketball, hockey, etc.)

- Activated during all-out exercise
- Produce much more lactic acid (compared with Type I) when activated
- Slow-twitch (Type I)
  - Predominantly aerobic fiber
  - Slow speed of contraction
  - Numerous large mitochondria
  - High level of enzymes
  - Especially good at metabolizing free fatty acids (FFAs)
  - Primary role is to sustain continuous endurance-type activities

Maximal O_2 Consumption:

This is the point at which the O_2 consumption plateaus and shows no further increase.

- Generally it is assumed that this represents the person's capacity for the aerobic synthesis of ATP.
- Any additional work accomplished is only done so by energy transfer of glycolysis (forming lactic acid).
- Oxygen consumption increases linearly with work intensity up to a point, beyond which an increase in work intensity will not elicit an increase in O_2 uptake.

Peak Vo_2:

Max Vo_2:

Max Vo_2 is defined as the maximal amount of oxygen one can consume in one minute and is reported in absolute terms as liters per minute or in relative terms as milliliters per kilogram of body weight per minute.

Max VO_2 is dependent on lung function, capacity, and diffusion; the heart and vascular system; blood volume; red blood cell (RBC) count; hemoglobin saturation; skeletal muscle type; capillary density; and mitochondrial function.

Cardiorespiratory fitness reflects the functional capabilities of the heart, blood vessels, blood, lungs, and muscles during exercise or physical activity.

Importance of Determining Cardiorespiratory Fitness:

- Prediction of certain medical conditions (e.g., low CRF associated with diseases such as cardiovascular disease, type 2 diabetes, metabolic syndrome, and certain types of cancers)
- Higher CRF is associated with decreased all-cause mortality.
- Skeletal muscle type, capillary density, and mitochondrial function

Chapter 4—Energy Transfer in Exercise   37

For Whom Is VO$_2$ Assessed?

- Athletes, especially endurance athletes

- General-population; individuals who are starting a wellness or fitness program

- High-risk individuals (pulmonary disease, heart disease, cancer, etc.). A person's CRF is often measured to see if certain treatment modalities are a viable option (e.g., transplants).

- Research participants

Difficulties with Assessing Max VO$_2$:

- More than 40% of healthy individuals have difficulty attaining a plateau in VO$_2$ during a maximal test.

- It is very difficult, if not impossible, for patients with cardiovascular or pulmonary disease.

- Many people interpret muscular fatigue as pain and cannot or will not continue to exercise until exhaustion.

- Exercising to maximal exertion can increase for untoward events (e.g., cardiac events).

- The risk of death during or immediately after an exercise test is less than or equal to 0.01% (1 in 10,000).

- The risk of acute MI during or immediately after an exercise test is less than or equal to 0.04% (4 in 10,000).

- The risk of a complication requiring hospitalization (including acute MI and/or serious arrhythmias) is less than or equal to 0.2% (2 in 1,000).

How Is Max VO$_2$ Measured?

- CRF can be measured or predicted using many methods.

- Best measurement of CRF involves maximal exertion, along with collection of expired gases for determination of MaxVO$_2$ (open- or closed-circuit spirometry).

- In open-circuit spirometry, oxygen consumption is determined by analyzing oxygen (O$_2$) and carbon dioxide (CO$_2$) concentrations during inspiration and expiration of air.

- In the development of an exercise prescription for the general population that is starting an exercise program, the Max VO$_2$ is often:

Estimated:
Predicted:

Understanding and measuring the relationship between the work of the cardio-vascular system (heart rate) and the amount of work being performed (work set on exercise testing device) is essential for predicting CRF.

CV Responses to Exercise:

•

If multiple submaximal HR/workload ratios are known, the maximal workload and consequently Max VO_2 can be determined by calculating the slope of the HR and VO_2 relationship and estimating the maximal HR.

Standard linear regression equation in which $y = mx + b$

> $y = VO_2$ variable
>
> x = HR variable
>
> m = slope
>
> Slope $(m) = (VO_2 2 - VO_2 1)/(HR2 - HR1)$
>
> $VO_2 1$ = Submax predicted VO_2 from stage 1
>
> $VO_2 2$ = Submax predicted VO_2 from stage 2
>
> HR1 = HR from stage 1
>
> HR2 = HR from stage 2
>
> Max VO_2 =

Instead of calculating the predicted Max VO_2, plotting the submaximal HR and VO_2 data graphically can be performed allowing the slope of the HR – VO_2 to be extrapolated to the age-predicted Max HR.

Sources of error in estimating and predicting Max VO_2:

- Prediction of HR_{max} by age
- Efficiency of the client on cycle ergometer or other testing equipment
- Calibration of cycle ergometer
- Accurate measurement of HR during each stage
- Having a steady state heart rate (HRSS) at each stage
- Not achieving a SVmax to provide a linear relationship between HR and exercise (typically HR < 120 bpm)

Factors to consider for selecting a CRF test:

- Time demands
- Expense or costs
- Personnel needed
- Equipment and facilities needed
- Physician supervision needed

Chapter 4—Energy Transfer in Exercise   39

- Population tested
- Importance of accuracy

What are the advantages of using submaximal tests?

What are the disadvantages of using submaximal tests?

Ergometry is the measurement of work output during a standardized work or exercise test.

The ability to determine or calculate the exact **work** output on an ergometer is essential for an exercise physiologist.

Work output (kp.m.min-1) = Resistance (kp) · Revolutions per minute (rpm) · Flywheel travel distance [meters per revolution (m · rev -1)]

Resistance is on flywheel by pendulum weight and friction belt measured in kiloponds (kp) or kilograms (kg)

The "standard" cadence for exercise testing is 50 rpm.

It may be adjusted to account for differences in fitness level or familiarity with cycling exercise.

For the flywheel to travel 50 rpm, a metronome for leg cadence would be set at 100 (one for each downward stroke of the leg).

Tachometer reading would be 18 km.hr-1

Example Work Outputs:

Watts are a more scientific unit of power and are frequently used in medical settings.

Watts can be determined from kp. m.min-1 by dividing by 6.1. In most instances this is approximated by dividing by 6.

For example, 600 kp. m.min-1 is approximately 100 watts (W).

Cycle Ergometry:

- Advantages

- Disadvantages

General Procedures for Submax Bike Test

- Position client on the bike. Adjust seat height to achieve 5° bend in knee at maximal extension. Adjust handlebars.
- Warm up at low intensity for 2–3 minutes.

- In 3-minute stages, HR should be monitored at end of 2nd and 3rd minute.

- Steady state should be achieved by end of stage. (If HR is > 110 bpm, two measures of HR should be within 6 bpm.)

- BP should be monitored at latter portion of each stage.

- RPE should be monitored at latter portion of each stage.

- Client appearance and symptoms should be monitored regularly.

- Test should be terminated when subject reaches 85% of age-predicted HR_{max} or 70% of HRR_{max}.

- Appropriate cool-down should be initiated.

- Continue all physiologic observations (HR, BP, signs and symptoms) for at least 4 minutes of recovery.

Balke-Ware Treadmill Protocol:

- 1-minute stages with relatively small MET increases between stages.

- Very useful for the development of the exercise prescription in clinical populations.

- Small MET increases allow tester to determine what intensity evokes symptoms (e.g., angina, ECG changes, O_2 desaturation, etc.).

- In the prescription, intensity is set slightly below the intensity that resulted in the onset of symptoms (e.g., HR 10–20 bpm below onset of angina /ECG changes).

Field Tests

- There are two common field tests that use a walking or running task to predict aerobic capacity:

- Rockport 1-mile walk test (submaximal)

- Cooper 1.5-mile walk/run test (maximal) or 12-min. run test.

- Less common: George jog test (submaximal)

Rockport Test:

Test may be useful for those who are unable to run or those with no more than moderate risk interested in starting a moderate, self-directed exercise program.

- Warm-up properly for brisk walking.

- Walk 1 mile briskly (HR > 120 bpm) around a measured course maintaining a relatively even pace

- Count recovery HR for 15 seconds immediately upon finishing the 1-mile walk.
Record 1-minute HR.

- Time is recorded in minutes and hundredths of a minute.

- VO_{2max} is calculated by the formula:

Chapter 4—Energy Transfer in Exercise   41

- $VO_{2max} =$

- Client should be able to walk briskly (get the exercise HR above 120 bpm).

- Client must NOT break into a run (one foot must make contact with the ground at all times).

- The formula is gender specific (the constant 6.315 is added to the formula for men only).

- The formula was derived from apparently healthy individuals ranging in age from 30 to 69. (r = 0.93, SEE 0.325L/min).

- Recently, a regression formula was created for college-age participants. VO_{2max} (ml/kg/min) = 88.768 + (8.892 for men) – (weight*0.2109) – (walk time*1.4537) – (HR*0.1194). (r = 0.84, SEE 0.389l/min).

Cooper Test:

Test is contraindicated for unconditioned beginners, individuals with symptoms of heart disease, and those with known heart disease or risk factors for heart disease.

- Warm-up properly for a maximal run.

- Run as fast as possible with even pacing for 1.5 miles (6 laps of a quarter mile or 400-meter track).

- Client is given feedback to help with even pacing.

- Time is recorded in minutes and hundredths of a minute.

- VO_{2max} is calculated by the formula:

A variation of the 1.5-mile run test is the 12-minute walk/run test. This test requires the client to cover the maximum distance in 12 minutes by either walking or running, or using a combination of both. The distance covered needs to be accurately measured and expressed in meters (to the nearest 50 meters).

George Jog Test:

- A submaximal 1-mile jogging test is an alternative to the maximal Cooper run test.

- Typical population assessed = fairly fit college-age persons.

- Jog 1 mile at a slow to moderate steady pace (men = 8 min. per mile; women = 9 min. per mile).

- Measure heart rate immediately upon completion of the 1-mile mark.

- Record time to the closest second.

$VO_{2max} =$

Maximal Exertion Protocols for Max VO$_2$:

Max VO$_2$ tests are utilized for many reasons:

Although complications with exercise testing appear to be low, a high degree of safety depends upon:

- Knowing when not to perform the test
- Knowing when to terminate the test
- Being prepared for any emergency

Additional Standardized Protocol:

- Ramping protocols
  - TM: Workload (speed or grade) increases approximately every 20 sec.
    - Ball State/Bruce TM ramp protocol
  - Bike: Watts increase at regular intervals depending upon the desired watts/min
    - 10–20 watts per minute ramp protocol

Max VO$_2$ Protocols:

- Taylor's Max VO$_2$ Test
  - 7.0 mph @ 2.5%, 5.0%, 7.5%, or greater
  - Test performed on consecutive days
  - Testing is complete when VO$_2$ increases by less than 2.5 ml/kg from one workload to the next
- Bruce. Max VO$_2$ Test
  - Exercise is performed on a treadmill. The test starts at 1.7 mph and at a grade (or incline) of 10%.
  - Percent grade can be modified to start at 0% then 5% for Stages 1 and 2.
  - At 3-minute intervals the incline of the treadmill increases by 2%, and the speed increases to 2.5, 3.4, 4.2, 5.0, then an increase of 0.5 mph and a 2% incline every 3 minutes.

Prediction of Maximal Aerobic Capacity from the Bruce Protocol:

- Three common approaches to predicting CRF from the Bruce protocol results:
  - Multiplication of the total test time
  - Prediction equation using the total test time cubed
  - MET cost estimates for each minute of the Bruce protocol

Chapter 4—Energy Transfer in Exercise   43

Oxygen Consumption During Recovery:

- After exercise, bodily functions and processes do not immediately return to resting levels.

- The time course of recovery depends on the intensity of exercise.

- O_2 Debt (EPOC): The oxygen consumed in excess of the resting value after exercise.

- Fast Component: If exercise was almost all aerobic, 1/2 of the total recovery O_2 consumption is repaid within 30 seconds. The remaining O_2 consumption is completed within several minutes.

- Slow Component: In recovery from strenuous exercise where lactic acid and body temperature increase significantly, O_2 consumption may remain elevated for several hours or even a day.

Possible Reasons for the EPOC:

- Body temperature can remain elevated after strenuous exercise, which can have a direct stimulating effect on metabolism, increasing O_2 consumption.

- As much as 10% of O_2 consumption goes to reload the blood from exercising muscles.

- 2%–5% goes to O_2 dissolved in body tissues and myoglobin.

- Must supply the respiring muscles and heart with O_2 after strenuous exercise.

- Tissue repair and redistribution of ions.

- Residual effects of hormones (e.g., epinephrine, norepinephrine, thyroxine, and glucocorticoids).

- The EPOC debt reflects both the anaerobic metabolism of exercise and the respiratory, circulatory, hormonal, ionic, and thermal adjustments that occur in recovery.

- This information is important when considering the time needed to recover from aerobic versus anaerobic (e.g., difference between long-distance running vs. sports such as basketball, hockey, soccer, tennis, etc.).

Review Questions: Chapter 4

(For true and false questions that are false, indicate what would make the question true)

1. The contributions from the various pathways of energy transfer depend upon:

   a. intensity of exercise

   b. duration of exercise

   c. fitness level of individual

   d. a and b only

   e. a, b, and c

2. An athlete sprints for 5–8 seconds. What energy system is the athlete primarily using?

3. If the athlete in question 2 sustains this effort, what energy system replenishes the ATP? This process results in the production of what important molecule?

   a. anaerobic glycolysis; lactic acid

   b. anaerobic glycolysis; pyruvic acid

   c. aerobic glycolysis; lactic acid

   d. aerobic glycolysis; pyruvic acid

4. When does blood lactate accumulate and rise in an exponential fashion in a healthy, untrained adult?

   a. at about 35% of maximal capacity for aerobic metabolism

   b. at about 55% of maximal capacity for aerobic metabolism

   c. at about 75% of maximal capacity for aerobic metabolism

   d. at about 95% of maximal capacity for aerobic metabolism

5. What will cause an increase in the blood lactate threshold?

   a. genetic endowment (type of muscle fiber)

   b. increased capillary density

   c. increased number and size of mitochondria

   d. increase in aerobic enzymes and transfer agents

   e. all of the above

6. *True or False:*

   Untrained individuals will reach a steady state of O_2 consumption more rapidly than trained individuals.

7. How does one know when a person is exercising at his or her maximal oxygen consumption?

   a. O_2 consumption will reach high values.

   b. O_2 consumption will plateau and show no further increase.

   c. O_2 consumption will continue to increase.

   d. O_2 consumption will increase rapidly.

Chapter 4—Energy Transfer in Exercise   45

Choose the characteristics that apply for the muscle fiber type.

8. Type II (fast-twitch muscle fibers) have the following characteristics:

    I. Possess a high capability for anaerobic production of ATP during glycolysis

    II. Especially good at metabolizing FFAs (free fatty acids)

    III. Activated during all-out exercises

    IV. Produce much more lactic acid

    a. I only

    b. II only

    c. IV only

    d. I and IV

    e. I, III, and IV

9. Type I (slow-twitch muscle fibers) have the following characteristics:

    I. Slow speed of contraction

    II. Numerous, large mitochondria

    III. Especially good at metabolizing FFAs (free fatty acids)

    IV. Primary role is to sustain continuous-endurance types of activities

    a. IV only

    b. I and IV

    c. I, II, III, IV

    d. none of the above

10. Define O_2 debt.

11. *True or False*:

    If exercise was almost all aerobic, 1/2 of the total recovery O_2 consumption is repaid within 30 seconds.

12. What is the main source for reestablishing glycogen levels after exercise?

    a. re-synthesized lactic acid

    b. protein in the diet

    c. carbohydrates in the diet

    d. fat in the diet

    e. b and c

13. *True or False*:

    Passive recovery will facilitate more lactate removal than moderate aerobic recovery.

14. What is a benefit of interval training?

    a. the overload of specific energy systems without too much lactate accumulation

    b. allows a greater duration of exercise and distance covered

    c. allows greater lactate accumulation

    d. a and b

15. List four difficulties with assessing Max VO_2.

16. Open circuit spirometry is often utilized:

    a. when a precise cardiopulmonary response to a specific therapeutic intervention is required.

    b. when the etiology of exercise limitation or dyspnea is known.

    c. when assisting in the development of an appropriate exercise prescription for cardiac and/or pulmonary rehabilitation.

    d. a and c

    e. all of these

17. *True or False:*

    An **estimated Max VO₂** is predicted from submaximal tests with either direct analysis of oxygen consumption or from the relationship between HR response and rate of work.

18. *True or False:*

    HR increases linearly with increasing aerobic exercise after SV reaches its maximal level.

19. List four sources of error in estimating and predicting Max VO_2.

20. Advantages of using a submaximal exercise test include which of the following?

    a. It's relatively inexpensive and requires less equipment, personnel, and medical supervision.

    b. The tests are generally shorter and easier to perform for the individual.

    c. It is an excellent way to diagnose medical problems.

    d. a and b

    e. all of these

5
Measurement of Energy Expenditure

Direct or Indirect Calorimetry:

- Direct:

- Indirect:

Two Ways to Measure Indirect Calorimetry:

- Closed-Circuit Spirometry: Used in resting studies, but not exercise studies because of the resistance in the circuit to moving large breathing volumes and because the production of CO_2 exceeds the rate at which it can be removed by the soda lime absorbent.

CRF Assessment with Open-Circuit Spirometry:

- By measuring a person's oxygen uptake, it is possible to obtain an indirect estimate of energy expenditure.

- Open-circuit spirometry is the most widely used technique to measure oxygen uptake, especially during exercise.

- In open-circuit spirometry, oxygen consumption is determined by analyzing oxygen (O_2) and carbon dioxide (CO_2) concentrations during inspiration and expiration of air.

Examples of Open-Circuit Spirometry:

- Portable Spirometer: Calculates volume of air flow, collects a small sample.

- Douglas Bag: A small sample of expired air is collected and then analyzed for its O_2 and CO_2 content.

- Situations in which open-circuit spirometry is appropriate include:

  - When a precise cardiopulmonary response to a specific therapeutic intervention is required

- When the etiology of exercise limitation or dyspnea is uncertain
- When evaluation of exercise capacity in patients with heart failure is used to assist in the estimation of prognosis and assess the need for transplantation
- When a precise cardiopulmonary response is needed within a research context
- When assisting in the development of an appropriate exercise prescription for cardiac and/or pulmonary rehabilitation

Oxygen Consumption Determination:

- Determine the amount of oxygen inspired (VOI).
- Determine the amount of oxygen expired (VOE).
- Subtract the expired oxygen from the inspired oxygen (VOI – VOE).
- The difference had to have been consumed (VO_2)
- The composition of inspired air remains relatively constant ($FiCO_2$ = 0.03% + FiO_2 = 20.93% + N_2 = 79.04%)
- It is possible to determine how much oxygen has been removed from the inspired air by measuring the amount and composition of the expired air.
- Expired air will have a 2.5–5.0% concentration of CO_2 ($FeCO_2$). Higher exercise intensity = Higher $FeCO_2$.
- Expired air will usually have a 15–18.5% concentration of O_2 (FeO_2). Higher exercise intensity = Lower FeO_2.
- $VO_2 = (Vi * FiO_2) – (VE * FeO_2)$, where Vi = volume of inspired air and VE = volume of expired air.

Gas Volumes During Physiologic Measurements:

- BTPS—Volume of a gas just as it is exhaled. Volume of a gas at body temperature, pressure, saturated.
- VATPS —Volume of a gas at ambient, temperature, pressure, saturated. Gas volumes measured during open-circuit spirometry are initially measured at ATPS.
- VSTPD—Volume of a gas after it has been standardized for temperature, pressure, and the effect of water vapor has been removed, or the gas has been dried.
- VO_2 can be affected by changes in pressure, temperature, and moisture content (H_2O vapor).
- Because at higher temperatures the number of water vapor molecules leaving the surface of a liquid increases, in order to maintain equilibrium (at saturation), it takes more water vapor to saturate the air, and thus the partial pressure is higher.

Open-Circuit Spirometry:

- VO_2 can be affected by changes in pressure, temperature, and moisture content (H_2O vapor).

- Therefore, VO_2 is most often reported as VSTPD, in that it is normalized to standard temperature (273 Kelvin), standard pressure (760 mmHg), and dry (correcting for the partial pressure of H_2O vapor).

Charles's Law

Temperature:

- Increasing the temperature increases the speed of the movement of the molecules, expanding the gas and increasing the volume proportionately.

Boyle's Law

Pressure:

- Increased pressure forces the molecules closer together, decreasing the volume proportionately to the increased pressure.

The volume of a gas varies depending on the amount of water vapor present.

The volume of the gas is greater when it is saturated with water than when the same gas is moisture free.

Even though the absolute number of molecules remains the same, the volume of a gas will vary depending on temperature, pressure, and water vapor.

Therefore, in order to be able to compare oxygen consumption in people tested in different environments, gas volumes must be standardized for temperature, pressure, and water vapor.

Standardize a Gas Volume for Temperature:

To reduce a gas to standard dry conditions, the effects of water vapor pressure at the ambient temperature must be subtracted from the volume of gas.

Because expired air is 100% saturated, it is not necessary to determine its % saturation from measures of relative humidity.

The vapor pressure can be found from a table. Look up the temperature and the pressure of the vapor, which is expressed in mmHg.

Respiratory Quotient (RQ):

- RQ is the ratio of metabolic gas exchange.

- Because of the inherent chemical differences in the composition of CHO, fats, and proteins, different amounts of O_2 are required to oxidize completely the carbon and H atoms in the molecule to form CO_2 and H_2O.

- Glucose:

- Fats (e.g., palmitic acid):

Chapter 5—Measurement of Energy Expenditure   51

- Protein:

- For most purposes, an RQ of 0.82 results from the metabolism of a mixture of 40% CHO and 60% fat.

- A measure of the gross (total) RQ is usually sufficient so that measurement of urinary nitrogen is unnecessary.

- Does exercise intensity and duration affect the measure of RQ?

Respiratory Exchange Ratio (RER):

- During steady-rate exercise, calculations of RQ are based on the assumption that the exchange of O_2 and CO_2 measured at the lungs reflects the actual gas exchange from nutrient metabolism in the cell.

- Respiratory Exchange Ratio: Term given when the exchange of O_2 and CO_2 at the lungs no longer reflects the oxidation of specific foods in the cells.

Examples:

- Hyperventilation:

- R can become > 1.0.

- Increase in VCO_2 without a similar increase in O_2 consumption.

- The increase in VCO_2 does not reflect an increase in oxidation of foodstuffs.

Exhaustive Exercise:

- $Hla + NaHCO3 \Leftrightarrow NaLa + H_2CO_3 \Leftrightarrow H_2O + CO_2 \Leftrightarrow$ Lungs

- This buffering process adds extra CO_2 to that quantity normally released during energy metabolism.

- R values in both cases can approach and be > 1.0.

- It is possible for R values to be < 0.7.

- After strenuous anaerobic exercise, CO_2 tends to be retained in the cells and body fluids to replenish the bicarbonate used to buffer lactic acid.

Caloric Equivalents of Foodstuffs Combusted Inside the Body:

Review Questions: Chapter 5

(For true and false questions that are false, indicate what would make the question true)

1. *True or False*:

   Direct calorimetry measures energy metabolism by measuring the O_2 consumption.

2. What are the percentages of O_2, CO_2, and N in ambient air?

   a. 79.04% O_2, 3% CO_2, 20.9% N

   b. 20.9% O_2, 3% $CO_2$2, 79.04% N

   c. 35.7% O_2, 0.03% CO_2, 79.04 N

   d. 20.9% O_2, 0.03% CO_2, 79.04% N

3. What does "RQ" stand for, and what is the equation used to obtain this number?

4. The RQ value is _____ for glucose, _____ for fats, and _____ for protein.

5. Why are RQ values different for the molecules in question 4?

6. Under what conditions can R become greater than 1.0?

   a. hyperventilation

   b. rest

   c. exhaustive exercise

   d. light aerobic exercise

   e. a and c

7. What is the purpose of a Douglas bag?

8. What is the definition of RER?

9. What is the mechanism that increases the RER during exhaustive exercise?

10. *True or False*:

    The measured RQ value would decline as the intensity of exercise increases.

11. List four situations for which open-circuit spirometry is appropriate.

12. _____ is the volume of a gas just as it is exhaled at body temperature, pressure, saturated.

    a. BTPS

    b. VATPS

    c. VSTPD

    d. VO_2

Chapter 5—Measurement of Energy Expenditure   53

13. a. VO_2 is most often reported as

    a. BTPS.

    b. VATPS.

    c. VSTPD.

    d. $FiCO_2$.

    b. Why is it primarily reported this way?

Chapters 4 & 5

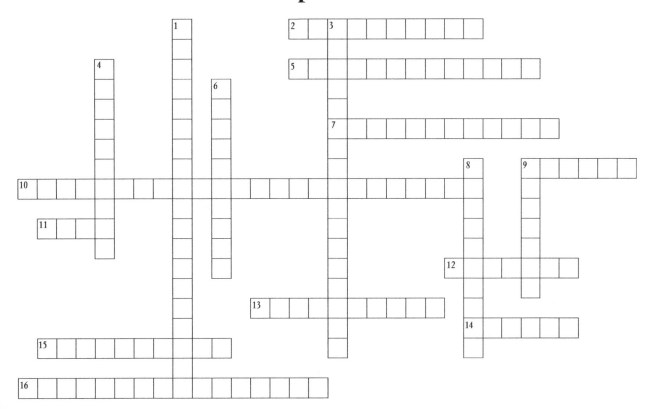

ACROSS

2 Type of fiber that generates primarily through aerobic pathways.
5 The difference between the total oxygen consumed during exercise and the total that would have been consumed during steady-rate aerobic metabolism.
7 The portion of the respiratory exchange attributed not to combustion of protein but only to carbohydrate and fat.
9 Abbreviated name for the immediate energy system.
10 The ratio of carbon dioxide produced to oxygen consumed.
11 Abbreviated term for recovery oxygen consumption.
12 The type of recovery that includes the individual laying down.
13 Name for the short-term energy system.
14 The type of recovery that includes performing submaximal exercise.
15 Total oxygen consumed in recovery minus the total oxygen theoretically consumed at rest.
16 Training that applies various work-to-rest intervals using super maximal exercise to overload the energy transfer systems.

DOWN

1 A guide to approximate the nutrient mixture catabolized for energy during rest and aerobic exercise.
3 Oxygen measured at the level of the lungs not at the active muscles.
4 Type of fiber that is active during change-of-pace and stop-and-go exercises.
6 Term for the plateau portion of the oxygen consumption curve.
8 Name for the rubber meteorological balloons used to measure expired air volume.
9 Name for the long-term energy system.

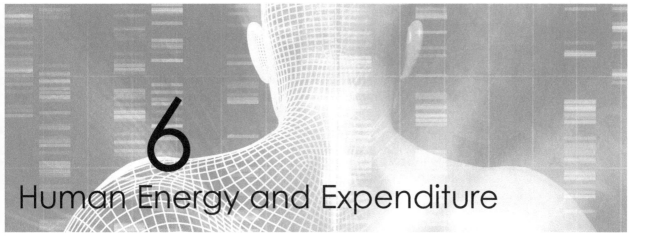

6
Human Energy and Expenditure

All chemical reactions in the body determine the body's metabolic rate and overall metabolism.

Total Daily Energy Expenditure (TDEE):

Basal Metabolic Rate:
- BMR is the minimum energy requirement to sustain the body's functions in the waking state.
- You can indirectly determine BMR by measuring resting oxygen consumption.
- A general estimate of BMR is body mass (kg) raised to the 0.75 power (body mass 0.75).
- BMR represents 60–75% of total energy expenditure in the average sedentary person.
- BMR is proportional to fat-free mass.
- On average, BMR decreases by 2–3% per decade.
- Physical activity may help to maintain BMR during weight loss by helping to maintain lean body mass.
- Limited data have shown that regular exercise (aerobic) may stimulate BMR through factors other than an increase in lean body mass.

Dietary-Induced Thermogenesis:
- Obligatory Thermogenesis: An increase in the energy metabolism attributable mainly to the energy-requiring processes of digesting, absorbing, and assimilating the various nutrients.
- Factors that can affect this include size of meal, macronutrient composition, elapsed time from meal, nutritional status, and health status.

- There is increased oxygen consumption after a meal due to digestion.
- Obligatory thermogenesis can account for 10–15% of our total energy expenditure.
- Facultative Thermogenesis: The activation of the sympathetic nervous system and the stimulator influence it may have on metabolic rate.

Energy Expenditure in Physical Activity:

- Expenditure depends on the intensity and duration of the physical activity.
- Energy expended during weight-bearing exercise increases in proportion to body mass.
- In non-weight-bearing activities (e.g., stationary cycling), there is little relationship between body mass and the energy cost of exercise.
- MET:
- MET represents an average person's resting metabolism or oxygen uptake.
- 1 MET = an oxygen uptake of 3.5 ml/kg/min.
- Using METs in determining an appropriate workload for exercising is simple, but first you must determine the maximal oxygen consumption.
- Treadmill (For walking, % grade unknown)
- Desired or known VO_2 = 3.5 + 2.68 (speed chosen) + 0.48 (speed chosen) (unknown % grade)
- Treadmill (For running speed unknown, 0% grade)
  - Known VO_2 = 3.5 + 5.36 (unknown speed) + 0.24 (unknown speed) (0 % grade)

- AirDyne (Unknown work level)
  - Known VO_2 = 3.5 + [2(unknown workload)/BW kg]
- StairMaster (Unknown setting)
  - Known VO_2 = 3.5(unknown machine setting)
- Stationary Bike (Unknown resistance)
  - Known VO_2 = 3.5 + [2(unknown resistance)/BW kg]
  - *Answer is given in kg·m·min^{-1}, and must be solved using the speed in pedal revolutions per minute and the distance the wheel travels per pedal revolution.
    - (Monark = 6 meters per complete pedal rev.)
    - Known kg-m-min = (unknown resistance in kg)(pedal revolutions) (6 meters per revolution)
- Concept II Rower (Unknown watts)
  - Known VO_2 = 3.5 + [2(unknown workload in kg-m-min)/Body Weight in kg]

Question: Cardiology sends you a patient with a VO_2 of 5 METs. At that workload, the patient starts to get chest pain (angina). The doctor wants him to exercise to build up his exercise tolerance while he assesses his treatment options. To keep him below the "angina threshold," you decide to exercise him at 80% of his symptom-limited Max VO_2. Calculate the MET level for this patient.

The Heart Rate Method:

- Established on the basis of the linear relationship between increasing workloads and heart rates.

- Based on the percentage of the maximal heart rate attained (the HR at the highest intensity achieved).

- Utilized because of the repeatable nature (given constant variables), and the reliability across all of the populations.

An estimation of the maximal HR can also be used, but this severely reduces the accuracy of pinpointing appropriate workloads in individuals who are prescribed medicines that slow the heart rate.

Karvonen Method:

- Used for determining Target HR utilizing the heart rate reserve (maximal HR minus the resting HR)

- Better for determining Target HR for people with resting heart rates outside the normal ranges (60–100), but is not limited to that population.

Sample Question: Using both the Karvonen method and a straight percentage method, calculate the target heart rate ranges at 80% of the maximum for a 20-year-old with a resting heart rate = 56 bpm.

Karvonen Versus Straight Percentage:

- Wide variation attained by using the two different formulas.

- Karvonen method uses more variables to lessen the impact caused by wide variations in the resting HR.

- More variables = specificity and individuality.

Percent HR Max.	Percent VO₂ Max.
50	28
60	42
70	56
80	70
90	83
100	100

Chapter 6—Human Energy and Expenditure   59

Sample Problem: You want your 42-year-old client to exercise at approximately 70% of her VO_2 max. If her resting heart rate is 72 bpm, what would be her target HR using the HR reserve (Karvonen) method?

The Challenge of Exercise Prescription in a Rehabilitation Setting:

- Medicines taken by individuals in a rehabilitative setting alter HR responses.

- Because these medicines alter the normal HR responses, the normal linear relationship between workload and heart rate **does not** exist. As a result, the psychological work that was discussed in the first lecture needs to be applied to any exercise testing or prescription.

Perceived Exertion Method:

- Utilization of this means of assessment assures the exercise physiologist that whether or not the normal physiological adaptations to activity are occurring, a method still remains to assess the amount of work being performed, leaving little risk of pushing the subject beyond his or her capabilities.

- The Borg Scale was designed to give a rough estimate of the percentage of maximal work performed during activity.

Sample Problem: A cardiac rehab patient graduates from Phase II and is referred to you by Cardiology to begin his Phase III program. His exit stress test from Phase II reveals a resting HR of 48 bpm and an exercise HR of 138 at a Perceived Exertion of 20 on a Borg Scale (suppressed because he is taking a beta blocker so his HR doesn't; go too high). His cardiologist says that he is cleared to exercise between the range of 70–80% of his Max HR. Determine his target HR zones and the appropriate Perceived Exertion number for 70–80%.

Duration of Activity:

- Intensity and duration have an inverse relationship.

  (As one increases, the other decreases to compensate.)

- ACSM recommendations for initial intensities:

Caloric Expenditure to Determine Duration Based on Fitness Level:

Category	Cal. Per Session
Low to Mid-Fair	100–200 kcal
Fair to Mid-Good	200–400 kcal
High	400+ kcal

Sample Problem: Using the formula (1 MET = 1 kcal/kg/hour), calculate the approximate caloric expenditure of a 128-pound female who exercises for an hour at an oxygen consumption of 38 ml/kg/min.

Oftentimes people do not realize that they have done too much until 24 to 48 hours later during the period of delayed onset muscle soreness (DOMS).

To lessen the possibility of exercising an individual "TOO HARD, TOO SOON," keep within the suggested caloric expenditure guideline standards for the three fitness groups outlined previously.

Remember, doing too much too soon is one of the major reasons for people dropping out of exercise programs.

Sample Problem: The female in the previous problem is 25 years old and falls within the AVERAGE fitness category (33–39 = Average). If the categories are LOW, FAIR, AVERAGE, GOOD, and HIGH, calculate the approximate amount of time she should exercise to burn the desired range of calories for her current fitness level.

Review Questions: Chapter 6

(For true and false questions that are false, indicate what would make the question true)

1. The three basic components of energy expenditure at rest are _____, _____ and _____.

   Matching:

   Match the next three questions with the term that best fits.

   a. Thermic effect of food

   b. Basal metabolic rate

   c. Dietary-induced thermogenesis

2. An increase in the energy metabolism attributed mainly to the energy requiring processes of digesting, absorbing, and assimilating the various nutrients. _____

3. The minimum energy requirements to sustain the body's functions in the waking state._____

4. Increased oxygen consumption after a meal due to digestion. _____

5. Which of the following characteristics apply to basal metabolic rate?

   I. Represents 60–75% of total energy expenditure in the average sedentary person

   II. Proportional to fat-free mass

   III. Represents 10–15% of total energy expenditure in the average sedentary person

   a. I only

   b. III only

   c. I and II

   d. II and III

6. *True or False:*

   Men and women have the same average rate of energy expenditure.

7. Tom and Jim ingest the same amount of calories, but differ in the amount of protein they ingest. Tom obtains 45% of his total calories from protein, whereas Jim obtains 10% of his total calories from protein. Which of the following is true?

   a. Tom and Jim will have a similar metabolic rate.

   b. Tom will have a higher metabolic rate due to a higher dietary-induced thermogenesis, which results from a higher protein intake.

   c. Jim will have a higher metabolic rate due to a higher dietary-induced thermogenesis, which results from a lower protein intake.

   d. none of the above

8. For every 1 liter of O_2 consumed, there are ____ kcal of energy expended.

9. ____ METs is equal to an oxygen uptake of ____ ml/kg/min.

Chapter 6—Human Energy and Expenditure   63

10. *True or False*:

    Acute exercise would significantly lower the diet-induced increase in caloric expenditure.

11. a. Define the Karvonen method.

    b. Use this method to calculate the target heart rate for a 47-year-old male whose resting HR is 83.

12. *True or False:*

    The percent of heart rate max is always higher than the percent of VO_2 max except at maximum capacity.

13. What are the ACSM recommendations for initial intensity and duration of exercise?

14. a. The normal caloric expenditure rate is approximately _____ of fat-free mass per hour during activity.

    b. If an individual has an initial fitness level classified as fair to mid-good, what is the target caloric expenditure per exercise session?

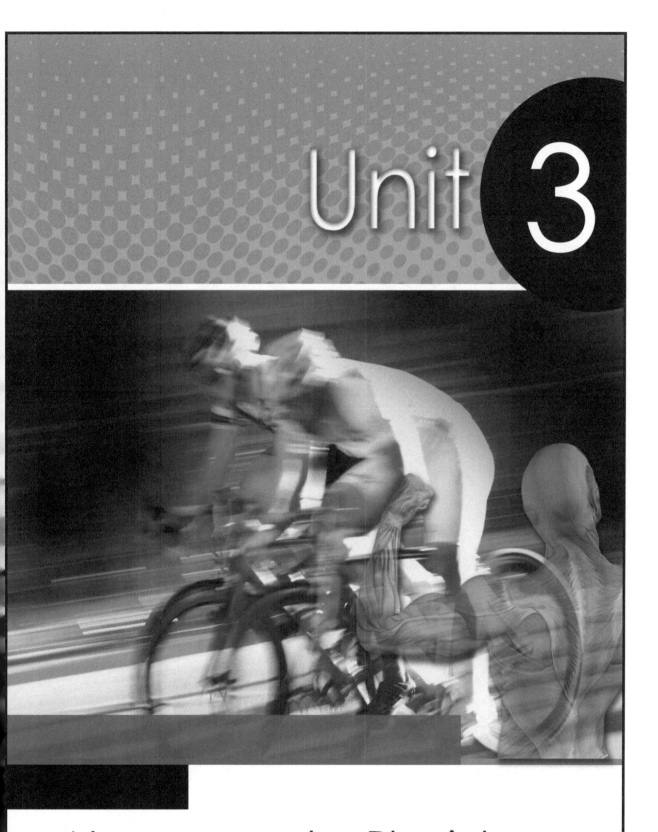

Unit 3

Neuromuscular Physiology and Exercise

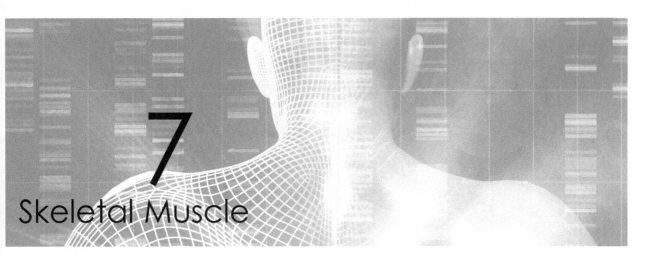

7
Skeletal Muscle

1. Neuromuscular system—coordination and integration of the muscles of the body together with the nerves that supply them.
2. Anatomy of a neuron
   a. Cell body (soma): dictates the critical firing rate of the action potential. Larger cell bodies are associated with higher critical firing rates. Also contain the structures involved in replication and transmission of the genetic code.
   b. Dendrites: short neural branches that receive impulses through numerous connections and conduct them toward the cell body.
   c. Axon: extends from the cell body to deliver action potentials toward the muscle to the motor endplate. Larger axons are associated with faster conduction velocities.
   d. Myelin sheath: a lipoprotein membrane that wraps around the axon over most of its length; acts as an electrical insulator that envelops the axon similar to the plastic coating around an electrical wire.
   e. Schwann cells: specialized cells that create or deposit the myelin sheath around the axon.
   f. Nodes of Ranvier: interrupt the myelin sheath every 1 to 2 mm along the length of the axon.
      i. The gaps or interruptions are uninsulated areas that allow the action potential to jump from node to node; this is known as saltatory conduction.
      ii. If no myelin were present, conduction velocities would be a lot slower.

g. Nerve terminal branches: multiple extensions of the axon that innervate individual muscle fibers.

h. Motor endplate or neuromuscular junction: represents the interface between the end of the axon at the terminal branch and the muscle fiber.

3. Macroscopic view of skeletal muscle

4. The skeletal muscles of the body are composed of multinucleated cylindrical cells called fibers, which run parallel to each other. Force is directed along the fiber's long axis.

5. Fiber length can vary from a few millimeters in the small muscles of the eye (i.e. ocular muscles) to approximately 30 cm in the large muscles of the leg (i.e. sartorius).

6. Connective tissue layers associated with skeletal muscle

a. Endomysium: a fine layer of connective tissue that wraps each muscle fiber and separates it from the neighboring fibers.

b. Perimysium: surrounds a bundle of up to 150 fibers.

c. Fasiculus: a large bundle of fibers.

d. Epimysium: a fascia of fibrous connective tissue that surrounds the entire muscle.

e. Tendons: dense connective tissue, the extension of the epimysium at the ends of the muscle.

f. Periosteum: bone's outermost covering; tendons connect the muscle to this covering of the bone.

7. Skeletal muscle structures

a. Sarcolemma: the muscle fiber membrane; a thin elastic membrane that encloses the fiber's cellular contents. The true fiber boundary.

b. Basement membrane: a loose collection of glycoproteins and collagen; outside the muscle fiber.

c. Sarcoplasm: contains the nuclei, substrates, and enzymes required for metabolism, the nuclei, mitochondria, and other specialized organelles.

d. Sarcoplasmic reticulum: highly specialized network of tubular channels that allows a wave of depolarization to spread rapidly from the sarcolemma to the inner environment through the T-tubules to initiate muscle contraction. Also stores a large concentration of calcium in the muscle fiber.

8. Myonuclei: true muscle fiber nuclei; muscle fibers are multinucleated; reside directly under the sarcolemma at the periphery of the fiber; represent 85 to 95% of the total nuclear pool.

   a. Myonuclear Domain Hypothesis

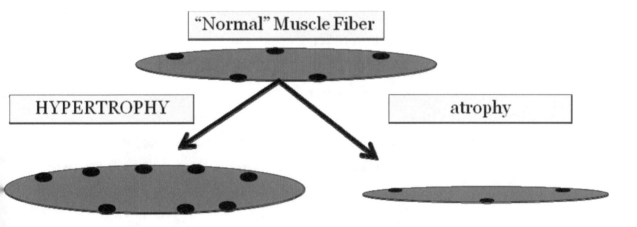

9. Satellite cells: lie between the basement membrane and the sarcolemma; these are quiescent myoblasts that function in muscle regeneration, muscle growth, exercise-induced adaptations, and recovery from injury.

   a. Upon activation

10. Skeletal muscle architecture

    a. Muscle origin: the location where the tendon joins a relatively stable skeletal part, generally the proximal end of the muscle.

    b. Muscle insertion: the location where the tendon joins a movable skeletal part, generally the distal end of the muscle.

    c. The force of muscle action transmits directly from the connective tissue, harness to the tendons, which then pull on the bone at the point of attachment.

11. Skeletal muscle fiber alignment: differences in fiber arrangement and length strongly affect a muscle's force and power generating capacity.

    a. Fusiform (spindle-shaped): the fibers run parallel to the muscle's long axis and taper at the tendon.

       i. Fiber length equals muscle length.

       ii. This fiber arrangement facilitates rapid muscle shortening.

b. Pennate (fan-shaped): fibers lie at angles, allow a large number of fibers into a smaller cross-sectional area; exhibit less range of motion.

  i. The degree of pennation directly impacts the number of fibers per cross-sectional area.

  ii. Allows individual muscle fibers to remain short; pennate muscles tend to generate considerable force and power.

  iii. Differ from fusiform muscles in three ways: contain shorter fibers; possess more individual fibers; exhibit less range of motion.

  iv. Unipennate muscle: soleus

  v. Bipennate muscle: rectus femoris

  vi. Multipennate muscle: deltoid

c. Other factors being equal, muscles with greater pennation, although slower in contraction velocity, generate greater force and power than fusiform muscles because more fibers contribute to the muscle action.

12. Composition of skeletal muscle

  a. Water—makes up approximately 75% of total muscle mass

  b. Protein—makes up approximately 20% of total muscle mass

  c. "Other"—makes up approximately 5% of total muscle mass

  i. High-energy phosphates (ATP)

  ii. Lactate

  iii. Minerals (calcium, magnesium)

  iv. Amino acids, carbohydrates, fats

  v. Enzymes

  vi. Ions (Na^+, K^+, Cl^-)

13. Blood supply to skeletal muscle: arteries and veins divide into numerous arterioles, capillaries, and venules to form a network in and around the endomysium.

  a. Role of blood supply to skeletal muscle:

  i. Numerous blood vessels supply the skeletal muscles to provide nutrients and oxygen, and to remove carbon dioxide and waste products.

  ii. Skeletal muscle oxygen uptake can increase up to 70× during intense endurance exercise. To increase blood flow during exercise, dormant capillaries are dilated.

    1. 200 to 500 capillaries deliver blood to each mm^2 of active muscle.

    2. Four capillaries contact each muscle fiber.

    3. With aerobic exercise training, the number of capillaries per muscle fiber may increase to 5 to 7 capillaries per fiber.

70   Chapter 7—Skeletal Muscle

Untrained Muscle
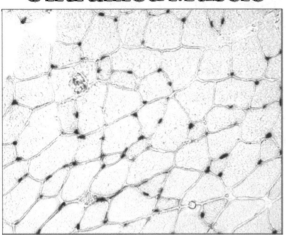

Trained Muscle
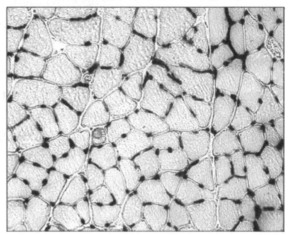

b. Effect of exercise on blood supply:

   i. Muscle contractions during endurance exercise

      1. Blood flow is reduced during active contractions.

      2. Blood flow increases during muscle relaxation.

      3. This provides a mechanism to move blood through the capillary bed of active muscles and propel it back to the heart.

      4. During intense or long-duration endurance exercise, the vascular bed delivers large quantities of blood through active tissues to accommodate the increased oxygen need.

      5. A trained muscle has an increased capillary-to-muscle fiber ratio. This is an indicator of oxidative potential of a muscle.

      6. The total number of capillaries per muscle averages 4% higher in endurance-trained athletes compared to untrained people.

      7. There is a positive relationship between VO_2max and the average number of muscle capillaries.

   ii. Muscle contractions during resistance exercise

      1. Local blood flow is occluded when a muscle generates 60% or more of its maximum force capacity due to increased intramuscular pressure.

      2. High-energy phosphates and glycolytic anaerobic reactions provide the main energy sources.

14. Myofibrils

    a. A single multinucleated muscle fiber contains myofibrils that lie parallel to the fiber's long axis.

15. Sarcomere—functional unit of the muscle fiber. The sarcomere consists of the basic repeating unit between two Z-lines.

    a. The sarcomere has a cross-striation pattern:

       i. Z-line: defines the sarcomere boundaries; adheres to the sarcolemma to provide stability.

ii. I-band: represents the light area of the sarcomere; contains actin only; there is no overlap of actin and myosin.

iii. A-band: represents the dark area of the sarcomere; this is due to the overlap of actin and myosin.

iv. H-zone: the center of the A-band; contains myosin only.

v. M-line: the center of the sarcomere; myosin filaments extend from the M-line.

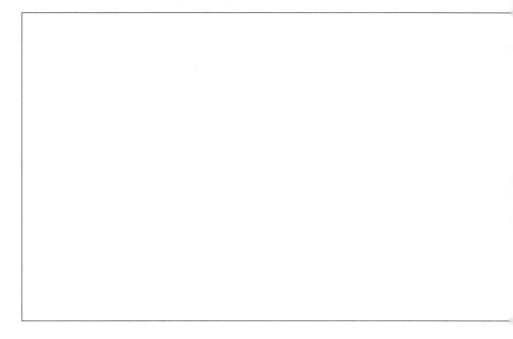

b. Sarcomeres in series: these are sarcomeres attached at adjacent Z-lines by the protein alpha-actinin.

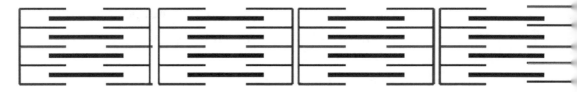

c. Sarcomeres in parallel: anchored at Z-lines by the protein desmin.

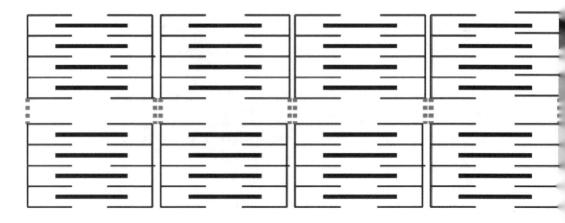

d. Comparison of sarcomeres in series and sarcomeres in parallel.

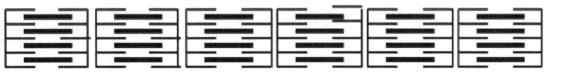

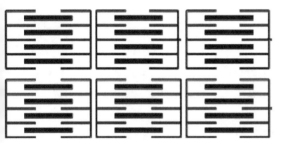

16. a. Contractile Proteins

    i. Actin: the thin filament; interacts with myosin.

    ii. Myosin: the thick filament; represents the motor protein of skeletal muscle; produces movement by the energy of ATP.

    b. Structural, costameric proteins

    i. Alpha-actin—approximately 7% of the Z-line protein; holds the actin filament in place spatially.

    ii. Desmin—forms connections between adjacent Z-lines from different sarcomeres; helps keep the sarcomere in register.

    iii. Titin: molecular spring.

    iv. Dystrophin: acts as a link between the outside and the inside of the muscle fiber through the formation of the dystrophin–glycoprotein complex.

    1. In the absence of dystrophin: the dystrophin–glycoportein complex does not form; this leaves the muscle fiber susceptible to contraction-induced ruptures; this leads to repeated cycles of muscle fiber degeneration and regeneration; this leads to the release of cytosolic components into the circulation.

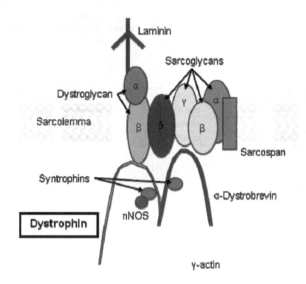

**Dystrophin Associated
Protein Complex (DAPC)**

    c. Regulatory contractile proteins

        i. Tropomyosin—covers the myosin-binding sites on actin; transduces the conformational change of the troponin complex to actin.

        ii. Troponin complex—located within the actin filament; acts as the switch that transforms the calcium signal into a molecular signal that induces cross-bridge cycling.

           1. Troponin-T:

           2. Troponin-C:

           3. Troponin-I:

17. Intramuscular network: a tubular system that functions to transport action potentials from the motor neuron to the muscle fiber.

    a. Transverse tubules (T-tubules): is an extension of the sarcolemma that lies transverse to the long fiber.

    b. Sarcoplasmic reticulum: stores calcium

        i. Terminal cisternae: the portion of the sarcoplasmic reticulum that is directly adjacent to a T-tubule.

        ii. Longitudinal portion: the portion of the sarcoplasmic reticulum that forms the large tubular network around the myofibrils.

c. Triad: a repeating pattern of two sarcoplasmic vesicles and T-tubule.

d. DHPR: dihydropyridine receptor, also known as the voltage sensor, converts the electrical action potential to a chemical signal.

e. Ryanodine receptor: the calcium release channel of the sarcoplasmic reticulum.

18. Neuromuscular junction (motor endplate): represents the interface between the end of a myelinated motor neuron and a muscle fiber.

a. Five characteristics of the neuromuscular junction:

   i. The presence of Schwann cells

   ii. The terminal branch of the neuron contains the neurotransmitter acetylcholine

   iii. A basement membrane that lines the synaptic space

   iv. A membrane opposite of the nerve terminal that contains acetylcholine receptors

   v. Connector microtubules at the postsynaptic membrane that transmit the electrical signal deep within the muscle fiber

b. Series of events at the neuromuscular junction:

   i. presynaptic membrane is depolarized

   ii. channels in the presynaptic membrane open, extracellular calcium enters the nerve terminal

   iii. Acetylcholine-containing vesicles fuse to the nerve terminal and release the acetylcholine via exocytosis

   iv. Acetylcholine is released into the synaptic space and binds to acetylcholine receptors in the postsynaptic membrane

   v. This depolarizes the postsynaptic membrane and leads to an excitatory postsynaptic potential (EPP)

   vi. The EPP, or action potential, propagates in all directions along the sarcolemma

   vii. Acetylcholinesterase in the synaptic space begins to degrade any acetylcholine that has not bound to a receptor

   viii. Choline, a by-product of that degradation, is taken back into the nerve terminal to be used to make more acetylcholine

19. Excitation–contraction coupling: in skeletal muscle, excitation–contraction (E–C) coupling describes a cascade of cellular events initiated by an action potential at the sarcolemma resulting in the release of intracellular calcium and ultimately muscle contraction.

a. Step 1: Generation of an action potential in the motor neuron causes the terminal axon to release acetylcholine which diffuses across the synaptic cleft and binds to specialized receptors on the sarcolemma.

Chapter 7—Skeletal Muscle   75

b. Step 2: The action potential is transmitted to the sarcolemma and spreads in both directions along the muscle fiber.

c. Step 3: The action potential enters the T-tubules and comes into contact with the DHPR, also known as the voltage sensor).

d. Step 4: The DHPR is physically coupled to the ryanodine receptor which acts as the Ca^{+2} release channel in the sarcoplasmic reticulum.

   i. The four monomers of the ryanodine receptor open allowing Ca^{+2} to leave the terminal cisternae portion of the sarcoplasmic reticulum due to the large concentration gradient.

   ii. Ca^{+2} is released in close proximity to the A–I band junction of the sarcomere.

e. Step 5: Ca^{+2} binds to troponin-C, causing tropomyosin to move and expose the myosin-binding sites on the actin filament. This movement is known as the tropomyosin shift.

76   Chapter 7—Skeletal Muscle

f. Step 6: Cross-bridge cycling begins and continues in the presence of Ca^{+2} (we will cover the myosin power stroke and the sliding filament theory in a subsequent section).

g. Step 7 (relaxation): there are several steps to initiate muscle relaxation following activation.

   i. Muscle stimulation from the efferent neuron stops; release of acetylcholine from the terminal branch stops.

   ii. The remaining acetylcholine in the synaptic space is completely degraded by acetylcholinesterase.

   iii. Ca^{+2} release from the sarcoplasmic reticulum stops.

   iv. The remaining Ca^{+2} is pumped back into the sarcoplasmic reticulum by sarcoplasmic endoplasmic reticulum calcium ATPase (SERCA) pumps.

   v. Tropomyosin moves back into its original orientation, covering the myosin binding sites on the actin filament inhibiting further interactions.

20. Sliding filament theory: proposes that a skeletal muscle shortens (concentric contraction) or lengthens (eccentric lengthening contraction) due to the thick and thin filaments sliding past each other without changing length.

   a. Force produced at Z-lines and the relative sizes of the zones within the sarcomere are altered:

      i. Concentric contraction: the I-band and H-zone decrease as the Z-lines are pulled toward the center of the sarcomere.

      ii. Isometric contraction: the fiber's length remains unchanged, so the relative spacing of the sarcomere remains the same.

      iii. Eccentric contraction: the A-band increases slightly as the fiber lengthens during an active contraction.

21. Actin and myosin interaction

   a. Myosin cross-bridges: globular myosin heads extend perpendicularly to latch onto the double-twisted actin strands to create structural and functional links between myofilaments.

   b. ATP hydrolysis activates the myosin heads, placing them in an optimal orientation to bind to actin.

   c. Myosin head:

      i. ATPase enzyme: myosin ATPase is located at the head of the myosin molecule; splits ATP and impacts the rate of muscular contraction.

   d. Myosin power stroke:

      i. State 1: resting position, ATP always bound at the head of myosin. There is no contact between myosin and actin in this state.

      ii. State 2: ATP is cleaved by myosin ATPase into ADP and inorganic phosphate (Pi). Myosin and actin are said to enter a "weakly bound state."

Chapter 7—Skeletal Muscle   77

iii. State 3: The Pi is released from its site on myosin; actin and myosin enter a "strongly bound state."

iv. State 4: The release of the ADP initiates the myosin power stroke; the myosin head swings approximately 60 degrees pulling the actin filament toward the center of the sarcomere. Actin and myosin will remain in State 4 until another ATP binds to myosin.

22. Length–tension relationship: is the isometric tension generated by the muscle at differing sarcomere lengths.

a. Optimal sarcomere length: maximal force occurs at this length.

b. In sarcomeres with lengths longer than optimal length, force output is lower due to fewer interactions of individual myosin heads with actin filaments.

c. In sarcomeres with lengths shorter than optimal length, force output is lower due to interference at the center of the sarcomere between opposing actin filaments.

23. Skeletal muscle fiber types: skeletal muscle contains two main types of fibers. These differ based on the primary mechanisms they use to

produce and use ATP, the type of motor neuron innervation, and the type of myosin heavy chain expressed.

a. The proportions of each type of muscle fiber vary from muscle to muscle and from person to person.

b. Type II (also known as fast, or fast-twitch fibers):

   i. Four characteristics contribute to this fiber's rapid energy generation for quick, powerful muscle actions.

      1. High capability for electronic transmission of action potentials

      2. Rapid calcium release and uptake by the *sarcoplasmic reticulum*

      3. High myosin ATPase activity

      4. High rate of cross-bridge turnover

   ii. The fast-twitch fiber's intrinsic speed of shortening and tension development ranges three to five times faster than slow-twitch fibers.

   iii. Fast-twitch fiber activation predominates in anaerobic-type sprint activities and other forceful muscle actions that rely almost entirely on anaerobic energy metabolism.

   iv. Activation of fast-twitch fibers plays an important role in the stop-and-go or change-of-pace sports such as basketball, soccer, lacrosse, and field hockey.

   v. Type II fibers distribute into three primary subtypes:

      1. Type IIa: represent the fast oxidative glycolytic fiber

      2. Type IIx: intermediate fiber

      3. Type IIb: possess the most anaerobic potential, most rapid shortening velocity, represents the true fast glycolytic fiber

c. Type I (also known as slow, or slow-twitch fibers)

   i. Four characteristics contribute to the slow fibers ability to generate energy through oxidative metabolism.

      1. Low myosin ATPase activity

      2. Slow calcium handling and shortening velocity

      3. Less well-developed glycolytic capacity when compared to Type II fibers

      4. Large and numerous mitochondria

   ii. Are highly fatigue resistant and ideally suited for prolonged aerobic exercise.

   iii. Both slow and fast fibers contribute during near maximum aerobic and anaerobic exercise

24. Basic fiber types based on twitch properties

   a. Fast glycolytic (FG)

   b. Fast oxidative glycolytic (FOG)

   c. Slow oxidative (SO)

Chapter 7—Skeletal Muscle   79

25. Basic fiber types based on myosin ATPase activity

26. Muscle contractile properties: determination of maximal force production, contraction velocity, and fatigue properties provide details about the myosin composition of a muscle and how a muscle handles calcium.

   a. Twitch contraction: a brief contractile response of a small number of muscle fibers within a muscle.

   b. Tetanus contraction: a maximal contraction of all the fibers within a muscle for a sustained period of time.

   c. Parameters obtained from a twitch contraction:

      i. Maximal force output (Pt)

      ii. Contraction time (CT) or Time to peak tension (TPT)

      iii. 1/2 relaxation time (1/2 RT)

   d. Tetanus contraction:

      i. Unfused tetanus

      ii. Fused tetanus

e. Differences in twitch and tetanus contractions when comparing fast and slow muscles.

27. Force–velocity relationship: describes the force that a muscle can generate at any given shortening velocity during concentric, isometric, and eccentric muscle actions.

a. Definitions/terms associated with this relationship

i. Muscle shortening: this area of the graph represents every shortening velocity which a muscle/muscle fiber can produce at any given force/resistance during a concentric contraction.

ii. Muscle lengthening: this area of the graph represents every shortening velocity which a muscle/muscle fiber can produce at any given force/resistance during an eccentric/lengthening contraction.

Chapter 7—Skeletal Muscle   81

iii. Vmax: is the maximal shortening velocity a muscle can produce against zero resistance.

iv. Isometric point (peak isometric force): this point represents the maximal weight at which no muscle shortening can occur. This is the intersection between the concentric and eccentric sections of the relationship.

v. 1 Repetition maximum (1RM): is the most weight that can be lifted for 1 repetition in any given resistance exercise.

b. How is the force-velocity relationship applied to exercise?

i. Concentric contractions at various percentages of 1RM

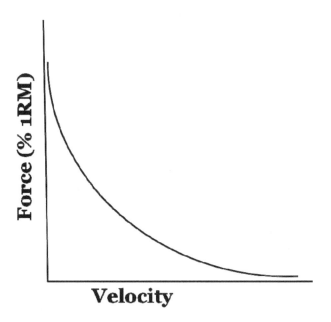

ii. Eccentric contractions at various percentages of 1RM

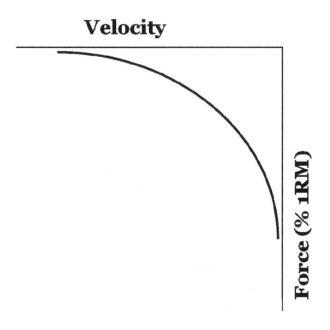

82 Chapter 7—Skeletal Muscle

c. Comparison of the force-velocity relationship in type II and type I muscle fibers

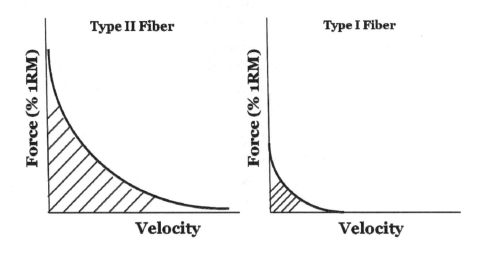

28. Power curves

   a. Power (P) = the rate at which work is performed, and is a product of the force-velocity relationship.

      i. P = Work/Time

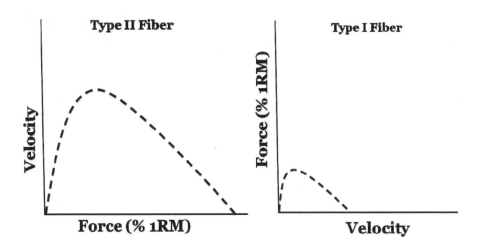

29. Performance characteristics and fiber type **(Table 7.1)**

   a. Fiber type transitions:

b. Untrained individuals on an average possess 45 to 55% slow fibers in the muscles of the arms and legs.
   i. While no gender differences exist in fiber-type distribution, there is a large inter-individual variation in fiber type.
   ii. Generally, the trend in one's muscle fiber–type distribution remains consistent among the body's major muscle groups.
c. Certain patterns of muscle fiber distribution appear when comparing highly-trained athletes
   i. Endurance athletes possess predominantly slow fibers.
   ii. Anaerobic athletes possess predominantly fast fibers.
   iii. Larger muscle fibers in male athletes and a larger total muscle mass are the main gender differences in muscle morphology.
   iv. Performance success is dependent not only on muscle fiber composition, but on a blending of many physiologic, biochemical, neurologic, and biomechanical support systems.
d. Effects of training

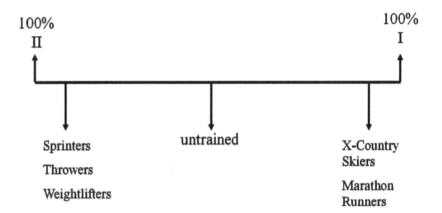

e. Fiber-type relationship to maximal oxygen consumption
   i. High VO$_2$max values typically associated with high type I fiber content
      1. Cross-country skiing: approximately 80% type I, 80 mL/kg/min
      2. 100 to 220 m sprinter: approximately 55% type I, 55 mL/kg/min
      3. Trained students: approximately 55% type I, 60 mL/kg/min

Review Questions: Chapter 7

(For true and false questions that are false, indicate what would make the question true)

1. Match the term with the appropriate definition:

    _____ perimysium   1. Fibrous connective tissue layer that surrounds entire muscle

    _____ fasciculus   2. The bone's outermost covering

    _____ epimysium   3. A bundle of approximately 150 muscle fibers

    _____ tendons   4. Connective tissue layer that surrounds a bundle of fibers

    _____ periosteum   5. Connects both ends of the muscle to the periosteum

2. The fixed or proximal end of the lever system, which is generally nearest the body's midline, where the tendon joins a relatively stable skeletal part is referred to as the _____.

3. The distal muscle attachment to a movable skeletal part is referred to as the _____.

4. Which of the following is in the correct order of innermost to outermost layers?

    A. endomysium, perimysium, epimysium

    B. fasciculus, endomysium, epimysium

    C. epimysium, fasciculus, endomysium

    D. epimysium, perimysium, endomysium

5. What protein is most abundant in the tendons?

    A. actin

    B. myosin

    C. elastin

    D. collagen

6. What are two roles of the sarcolemma?

    A. action potential conduction and structure

    B. structure and growth

    C. growth and action potential conduction

    D. metabolism and action potential conduction

7. Which is the most abundant protein within skeletal muscle?

    A. actin

    B. myosin

    C. tropomyosin

    D. titin

8. During intense muscle contractions, which is NOT a primary energy system used?

   A. oxidative phosphorylation

   B. ATP/CP

   C. slow glycolysis

   D. all of these would be used equally

9. What is the functional unit of a muscle fiber?

   A. myofibril

   B. sarcomere

   C. M-band

   D. motor unit

10. *True or False:*

    Overall, pennate muscles produce less force than fusiform muscles.

11. Which of the following muscle types typically has the greatest physiological cross-sectional area?

    A. smooth muscle

    B. fusiform muscle

    C. pennate muscle

    D. cardiac muscle

12. The transverse tubules (t-tubules) are responsible for transmitting which of the following?

    A. action potentials

    B. calcium ions

    C. ATP

    D. acetylcholine

13. *True or False:*

    The Sliding Filament Theory states that concentric muscle contractions are due to shortening of muscle fibers and eccentric contractions are due to lengthening of muscle fibers.

14. *True or False:*

    The Sliding Filament Theory states that actin and myosin filaments change length during a muscle contraction.

15. List the following events in the correct order.

    1. Calcium is released from the SR.

    2. Calcium binds to troponin-C.

    3. T-tubules transmit an action potential.

    4. Tropomyosin shift occurs.

    5. Muscle contraction occurs.

86   Chapter 7—Skeletal Muscle

6. Myosin power stroke occurs.

    A. 1, 2, 3, 4, 5, 6

    B. 3, 1, 2, 4, 6, 5

    C. 5, 3, 6, 1, 2, 3

    D. 2, 6, 1, 5, 3, 4

    E. 4, 5, 2, 3, 1, 6

16. Sam is a world-class sprinter. Which of the following are characteristics of the predominant muscle fiber type that would contribute to his ability (circle all that apply)?

    A. high myosin ATPase activity

    B. rapid calcium release and uptake by the SR

    C. high oxidative capacity

    D. high glycolytic capacity

    E. high resistance to fatigue

17. Jess, Sarah, and Katie are all runners. Jess never stretches and can't touch her toes. Sarah stretches moderately, and Katie stretches twice per day 7 days per week. All things being equal, whose muscles would produce the most force during an isometric contraction?

    A. Jess's

    B. Sarah's

    C. Katie's

    D. No differences would be observed; stretching does not affect muscle force

18. All of the following are subunits of the troponin complex EXCEPT:

    A. T.

    B. I.

    C. P.

    D. C.

19. In a skeletal muscle fiber, the myonuclei are located

    _____.

20. *True or False:*

A tetanus contraction is a maximal contraction of all the fibers within a muscle, and results in higher forces than a twitch contraction.

Chapter 7

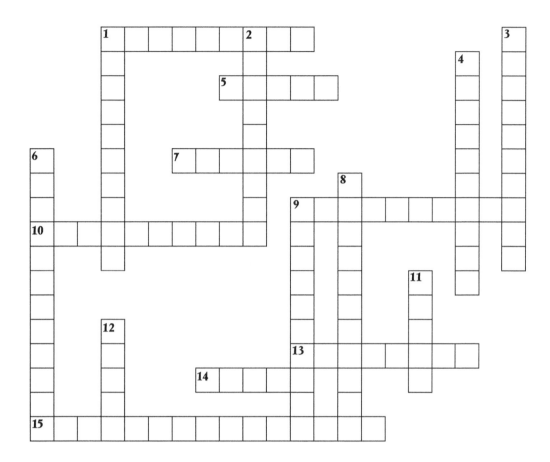

ACROSS

1. The functional unit of the muscle fiber.
5. Elastic filament that helps keep the thick filaments centered between two Z lines during contraction.
7. Thick filament, accounts for approximately 60% of muscle protein.
9. The layer of connective tissue that surrounds a bundle of up to 150 fibers.
10. The aqueous protoplasm that contains enzymes, fat and glycogen particles, nuclei, etc.
13. Protein that, in addition to calcium, triggers the myofibrils to interact and slide past each other.
14. Area of sarcomere containing only actin.
15. The model used to explain muscle contraction.

DOWN

1. Muscle fibers that generate energy for ATP resynthesis predominantly through the aerobic system of energy transfer.
2. A fascia of fibrous connective tissue that surrounds the entire muscle.
3. A thin elastic membrane that encloses the fiber's cellular contents.
4. Muscle fibers that exhibit high capability for electrochemical transmission of action potential.
6. Projections that spiral around the myosin filament in the region of overlap of actin and myosin filaments.
8. Protein that inhibits actin and myosin interaction.
9. The bone's outermost covering.
11. Area of sarcomere containing actin and myosin.
12. Area of sarcomere containing only myosin.

8
Neural Control of Human Movement

1. The nervous system: the effective application of force during complex learned movements depends on a series of coordinated neuromuscular patterns, not just on muscle strength.

2. The human nervous system consists of two major components.

   a. Central nervous system (CNS) consisting of the brain and spinal cord.

   b. Peripheral nervous system (PNS) consisting of nerves that transmit information to and from the central nervous system.

3. CNS: the brain

   a. Neural plasticity: brain cells, spinal neurons, neural circuits are created throughout life.

   b. Regular physical activity contributes to the development and maintenance of optimal brain function in middle and older age.

   c. The brain is divided into six main areas: medulla oblongata, pons, midbrain, cerebellum, diencephalon, telencephalon.

      i. The brain stem consists of the medulla oblongata, pons, and midbrain.

         1. Medulla oblongata: located immediately above the spinal cord and extends into the pons. Serves as a bridge between the two hemispheres of the cerebellum.

         2. Pons: part of the brain stem.

         3. Midbrain: only 1.5 cm long, attaches to the cerebellum and forms the connection between the pons and the cerebral hemispheres.

Chapter 8—Neural Control of Human Movement   91

4. The brain stem provides specialized control functions:

    a. Control of respiration

    b. Control of the cardiovascular system

    c. Control of the gastrointestinal system

    d. Control of many stereotyped movements of the body

    e. Control of equilibrium

    f. Control of eye movement

ii. Cerebellum: motor control center that provides fine tuning of muscle actions.

    1. Functions as the major comparing, evaluating, and integrating center for postural adjustments, locomotion, maintenance of equilibrium, perceptions of speed of body movement, and other diverse reflex functions related to movement.

    2. Consists of two peach-sized mounds of folded tissue with lateral hemispheres and a central lobe called the vermis.

iii. Diencephalon: located immediately above the midbrain and forms part of the cerebral hemispheres. The major structures include the thalamus, hypothalamus, epithalamus, and subthalamus.

iv. Telencephalon: contains the two hemispheres of the cerebral cortex, which makes up approximately 40% of the total brain weight. It is divided into four lobes— frontal, temporal, parietal, and occipital.

4. CNS: The spinal cord provides the major conduit for the two-way transmission of information from skin, joints, and muscles to the brain.

    a. Provides communication throughout the body via spinal nerves of the PNS).

    b. Contains three types of neurons

        i. motor neurons (efferent): provide communication with extrafusal and intrafusal fibers in skeletal muscle.

        ii. sensory neurons (afferent): provide communication from the periphery to the spinal cord.

        iii. interneurons

    c. Ascending nerve tracts: forward sensory information from peripheral receptors to the brain for processing. Three neurons form this sensory pathway:

        i. The axon of the cell body of the first neurons relays information to the spinal cord.

        ii. The cell body of the second neurons lies within the spinal cord.

iii. The axon of the third neuron passes up the central command center in the cerebral cortex.

iv. Sensory receptors serve as specialized receptors to detect conscious and subconscious information.

1. Conscious receptors show sensitivity to body position, temperature, and sensations of light, sound, small, taste, touch, and pain.

2. Subconscious receptors show changes in the body's internal environment:

a. chemoreceptors: respond to changes in blood gas tension and pH.

b. baroreceptors: react rapidly to changes in arterial blood pressure.

c. mechanoreceptors: react to mechanical stimuli such as touch, pressure, stretch, and motion.

d. Descending nerve tracts: axons from the brain move downward through the spinal cord along two major pathways:

i. pyramidal tract activates the skeletal musculature in voluntary movement under direct cortical control.

ii. extrapyramidal tract controls posture and muscle tone.

5. The PNS: contains nerves that transmit information to and from the central nervous system. It contains 31 pairs of spinal nerves and 12 pairs of cranial nerves.

a. Cranial nerves transmit sensory information and/or motor information.

b. Spinal nerves: consist of 8 pairs of cervical nerves, 12 pairs of thoracic nerves, 5 pairs of lumbar nerves, 5 pairs of sacral nerves, and 1 pair of coccygeal nerves.

c. Afferent neurons: relay sensory information from receptors in the periphery toward the central nervous system.

d. Efferent neurons: transmit information away from the central nervous system to peripheral tissues.

i. Somatic nerves (also called motor neurons): innervate skeletal muscles and produce an excitatory response in activated tissue.

ii. Autonomic nerves (also called visceral nerves or involuntary nerves): produce either an excitatory or inhibitory response; activate cardiac muscle, sweat and salivary glands, some endocrine glands, and smooth muscle cells in the intestines and walls of blood vessels. They can be divided into:

1. Sympathetic nervous system: sympathetic neurons emerge from the middle third of the spinal column (thoracic and lumbar segments) and supply the heart, smooth muscle, sweat glands, and viscera.

Chapter 8—Neural Control of Human Movement   93

2. Parasympathetic nervous system: parasympathetic neurons emerge from the brain stem and the lowest spinal cord segment and supply the thorax, abdomen, and pelvic regions.

6. Reflex arc:

    a. Afferent neurons enter the spinal cord through the dorsal root and transmit information from the peripheral receptors.

    b. These neurons synapse with the spinal cord through interneurons that relay information to different cord levels.

    c. The impulse then passes through the motor root pathway via anterior motor neurons to the peripheral organs (i.e. muscles).

7. Nerve supply to skeletal muscle: there are approximately 420,000 motor nerves that innervate approximately 250 million muscle fibers contained in the body.

    a. Motor unit: consists of the alpha motor neuron and all of the muscle fibers it innervates and is the functional unit of movement.

    b. Motor unit pool: the collection of the alpha motor neurons that innervate a muscle.

        i. Each muscle fiber receives input from one neuron, but a motor neuron may innervate many muscle fibers.

    c. One nerve or its terminal branches innervate at least one of the body's approximate 250 million muscle fibers.

        i. The number of muscle fibers per motor neuron generally relates to a muscle's particular movement function.

            1. A ratio of 1 neuron to 10 muscle fibers exists in the small muscles of the eye, and enables fine control of movement.

            2. A ratio of 1 neuron to 1600 muscle fibers exists in the gastrocnemius muscle and enables gross control of movement.

            3. The average ratio in the body is 1 neuron to 100/200 muscle fibers.

8. Excitation: occurs at the neuromuscular junction, produces an excitatory postsynaptic potential (EPSP).

    a. When the action potential arrives at the neuromuscular junction, acetylcholine is released from the terminal axon into the synaptic cleft and binds to acetylcholine receptors.

    b. The change in electrical properties elicits an end plate potential that spreads from the motor end plate to the sarcolemma on the muscle.

    c. This causes a wave of depolarization to travel the length of the fiber and into the T-tubule causing release of calcium.

    d. Acetylcholine is degraded within 5 minutes of its release by the enzyme acetylcholinesterase.

    e. Acetylcholine is resynthesized from acetic acid and choline, and repackaged into vesicles in the nerve terminal.

9. Inhibitory postsynaptic potential (IPSP)

   a. Some presynaptic neurons produce inhibitory impulses that increase the postsynaptic membrane permeability to potassium and chloride ions, thus decreasing the cell's resting membrane potential.

   b. IPSPs hyperpolarize the neuron making it more difficult to fire an impulse.

   c. Neural inhibition has protective functions and reduces the input of unwanted stimuli to produce a smooth purposeful response.

10. All or None principle: states that when the action potential is propagated along the axon and reaches the nerve terminal, all the muscle fibers that the nerve innervates will be stimulated and contract.

11. Motor unit functional characteristics: motor units are classified based upon the physiological and mechanical properties of the muscles they innervate. A motor unit contains only one specific muscle fiber type.

    a. Motor unit types:

       i. Fast-twitch fatigue sensitive (FF)

       ii. Fast-twitch fatigue resistant (FR)

       iii. Slow-twitch (S)

    b. Size principle: motor units are recruited in order, according to size, as a voluntary contraction increases from zero force to maximal voluntary force. Generally, larger motor units are activated in response to higher external loads, to produce greater forces.

       i. All motor units do not fire at the same time. It appears that smaller motor units are activated first as a result of their lower recruitment threshold while the larger motor units take longer to activate.

Chapter 8—Neural Control of Human Movement   95

12. Motor unit recruitment patterns: the nervous system has two primary mechanisms to vary a muscle's contractile force.

  a. Motor unit recruitment: is a process by which the nervous system activates additional motor units within a muscle.

  b. Rate coding: is a process by which the frequency of neural impulses conducted by activated motor neurons is increased.

    i. The upper limit of motor unit recruitment is achieved, rate coding is used to increase muscle force.

    ii. The discharge rate of motor units matches the fiber type, with type II fibers having a higher firing rate than type I.

13. Receptors of the muscles, joints, and tendons: sensory receptors in the muscles and tendons are sensitive to stretch, tension, and pressure. These receptors relay information about muscular dynamics and limb movement to conscious and subconscious portions of the nervous system.

This allows for continuous monitoring of the progress of any sequence of movements and serves to modify subsequent motor behavior.

  a. Muscle spindle: provides mechanosensory information about changes in muscle fiber length (i.e. stretch).

    i. Primarily respond to any stretch of a muscle and initiates a stronger muscle action to counteract this stretch.

    ii. The muscle spindle detects, responds to, and modulates changes in the length of muscle fibers to provide an important regulatory function for movement and maintenance of posture.

    iii. Three main components of the patella stretch reflex, as an example of muscle spindle activity:

      1. Muscle spindle senses and responds to the stretch.

      2. Afferent nerve fibers carry the sensory information from the spindle to the spinal cord.

      3. Efferent nerve fibers activate the stretch muscle fibers to contract harder.

  b. Golgi tendon organ (GTO): located in the region of the muscle where muscle fibers mesh with connective tissue in the tendon.

    i. The GTO detects differences in the tension generated by active muscle to protect the muscle and surrounding connective tissue from injury due to sudden or excessive loads.

    ii. When stimulated, the GTO transmits signals to the spinal cord to elicit a reflex inhibition of the muscle.

14. Neuromuscular fatigue: fatigue is the decline in muscle tension or force generating capacity in response to repeated stimulation during a given period of time.

  a. As muscle function changes during prolonged exercise, additional motor unit recruitment maintains force output as necessary, to maintain constant levels of performance.

  b. There are four main factors that relate to fatigue of voluntary muscle actions:

    i. CNS fatigue

    ii. PNS fatigue

    iii. Neuromuscular junction fatigue

    iv. Muscle fiber fatigue

      1. Creatine phosphate decrease

      2. Alterations in myosin ATPase

      3. Reduced metabolic enzyme activities

      4. T-tubule system fatigue

      5. Imbalances in ion concentrations

Review Questions: Chapter 8

(For true and false questions that are false, indicate what would make the question true)

1. Match the following parts of the brainstem with the correct description.

    1. midbrain

    2. medulla

    3. pons

        A. _____ serves as a bridge between the two hemispheres of the cerebellum

        B. _____ contains part of the extrapyramidal motor system

        C. _____ serves as a connection between the medulla and the midbrain

2. The cerebellum receives motor output signals from the _____ in the _____.

3. The peripheral nervous system contains _____ pairs of spinal nerves and _____ pairs of cranial nerves.

4. Match the number of pairs of spinal nerves to the specific area (numbers can be used more than once).

    A. _____ cervical   1. 14 pairs of nerves

    B. _____ thoracic   2. 5 pairs of nerves

    C. _____ lumbar   3. 8 pairs of nerves

    D. _____ sacral   4. 12 pairs of nerves

5. The peripheral nervous system contains both _____ neurons, which relay sensory information to the CNS, and _____ neurons, which transmit information from the brain to the peripheral muscles.

6. The autonomic nervous system is divided into the _____ and _____.

7. The central nervous system consists of

    A. the brain.

    B. the spinal cord.

    C. the nerves.

    D. all of the above.

    E. A and B.

8. What is the connection between the brain and the spinal cord?

    A. medulla oblongata

    B. pons

    C. brainstem

    D. cervical vertebrae

Chapter 8—Neural Control of Human Movement   99

9. The sensory division is also known as the _____ division and the motor division is also known as the _____ division.

    A. afferent; efferent

    B. efferent; afferent

    C. voluntary; involuntary

    D. involuntary; voluntary

10. Which body part has the fewest number of muscle fibers per motor neuron?

    A. leg

    B. eye

    C. fingers

    D. tongue

11. What is considered the functional unit of movement, consisting of an alpha motor neuron and its associated muscle fibers?

    A. motor unit

    B. reflex arch

    C. sarcomere

    D. fascicle

12. *True or False:*

Large somas have higher critical firing rates.

13. What is the main function of the phospholipid myelin sheath?

    A. insulates axons to preserve warmth

    B. protects the neuron

    C. speeds action potential transmission through saltitory conduction

    D. structurally supports the axon

14. *True or False:*

Each motor unit can only innervate one muscle fiber type.

15. Which ion(s) have a greater intracellular concentration across the neuron membrane?

    A. sodium

    B. chloride

    C. potassium

    D. A and B

    E. all of the above

16. What describes an increase in frequency of action potentials from activated motor neurons?

    A. motor unit recruitment

    B. rate coding

    C. temporal summation

    D. spatial summation

17. Which motor unit type is the last to fire during a muscle contraction?

    A. slow-twitch

    B. fast-twitch fatigue resistant

    C. fast-twitch fatigue sensitive

    D. these will all be recruited at the same time

18. *True or False:*

    Small somas have high critical firing rates and are associated with endurance activities.

19. Which of the following does NOT contribute to neuromuscular fatigue?

    A. alterations in levels of neurotransmitters

    B. accumulation of glycogen

    C. accumulation of lactate

    D. fatigue at the neuromuscular junction

20. Muscle spindles sense:

    A. fiber length.

    B. fiber strength.

    C. both C and D.

    D. none of the above.

21. What does the golgi tendon organ provide protection against?

    A. sudden or excessive load

    B. excessive stretch

    C. neuromuscular fatigue

    D. obesity

22. What part of the brain monitors and controls movement?

    A. brainstem

    B. parietal lobe

    C. pons

    D. cerebellum

23. What is a consequence of an inhibitory postsynaptic potential?

    A. polarization

    B. depolarization

    C. repolarization

    D. hyperpolarization

24. What is the point at which a nerve innervates a muscle?

    A. motor endplate

    B. neuromuscular junction

    C. motor unit

    D. A and B

    E. B and C

25. When a motor neuron is activated, what muscle fibers in the motor unit contract?

    A. all of them, synchronously

    B. it depends on the strength of the action potential

    C. all of them, starting with the slow oxidative fibers followed by the fast fibers

    D. it depends on the length of the action potential

Chapter 8

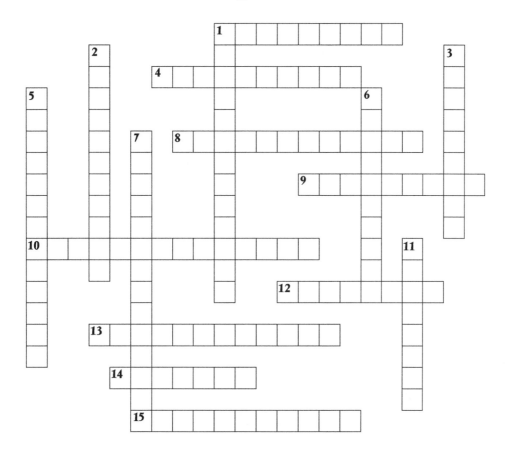

ACROSS

1 Consists of the medulla, pons and midbrain.
4 Thin outer membrane that covers the myelin sheath.
8 Lipoprotein membrane that wraps around the axon over most of its length.
9 Defines the skin area innervated by the dorsal roots of a single spinal segment.
10 Accounts for 40% of total brain weight and houses neurons for sensory and motor functions.
12 Types of sensory nerve fibers that enter the spinal cord by way of the dorsal horn.
13 Regulates metabolic rate and body temperature.
14 Nerve fibers that innervate skeletal muscle.
15 Specialized cell that covers the bare axon and then spirals around it.

DOWN

1 Receptors that react rapidly to changes in arterial blood pressure.
2 Collection on CNS axons.
3 Nerve fibers that activate cardiac muscle, sweat and salivary glands and some endocrine glands.
5 Region for neural impulse transmission between nerve and muscle fiber.
6 Collection of neuronal cell bodies in the CNS.
7 Receptors that respond to changes in blood gas tension and pH.
11 Collection of neurons in the peripheral nervous system.

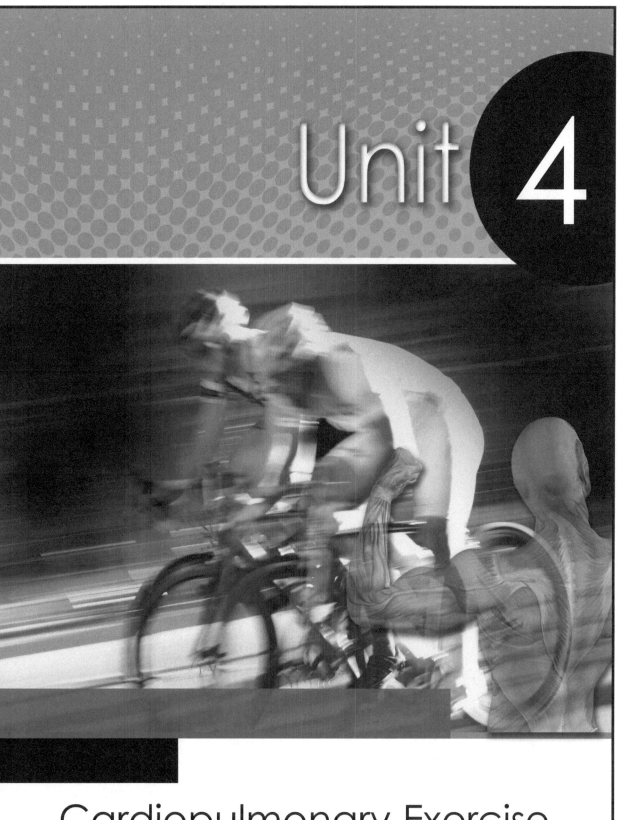

Unit 4

Cardiopulmonary Exercise Physiology

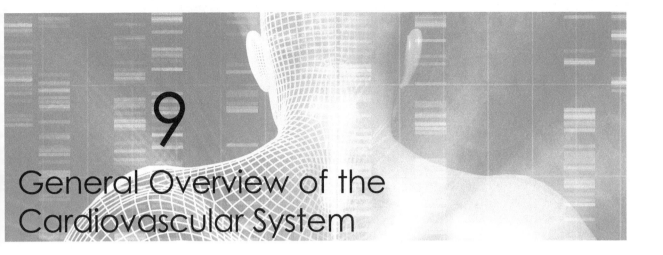

General Overview of the Cardiovascular System

Five IMPORTANT Functions of the Cardiovascular (CV) System

- Delivers _____ to active tissues
- Returns _____ blood to the lungs
- Transports _____, a by-product of cellular metabolism, from the body's core to the skin
- Delivers _____, _____ to active tissues
- Transports _____, the body's chemical messengers

Circulatory System

- The heart is a dual pump.
- Two blood flow circuits:
    - **pulmonary circulation**—between the heart and lungs
    - **systemic circulation**—between the heart and other body systems

Systemic circulation is the portion of the CV which carries _____ blood away from the heart, to the _____, and returns _____ blood back to the heart.

Pulmonary circulation is the portion of the CV which carries _____ blood away from the heart, to the _____, and returns _____ blood back to the heart.

The heart's only function is to pump blood.

Change in Left Ventricular Mass

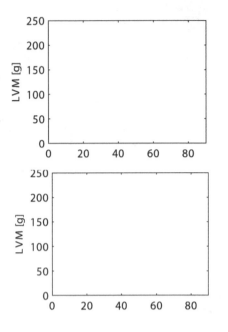
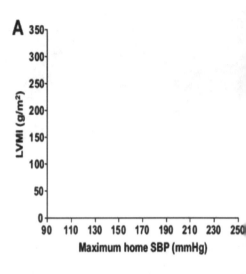

Heart Valves

- Blood flows through the heart in one direction—from veins, to atria, to ventricles, to arteries.
- Heart valves ensure that blood flows in the right direction through the heart.
- Valves are positioned so that they open and close passively because of pressure differences.

Filling of the Ventricles

Passive filling of the ventricles is governed by _____ gradients.

Active filling—atrial contraction _____

- At resting heart rates, the atrial contraction only contributes _____ % to the filling of the ventricle

Approximately 70% of the venous return (blood returning to the heart) enters the ventricles before the atria undergo contraction

Heart Contraction

Isovolumetric Contraction

For a brief period of time (_____ to _____ sec), when all heart values remain shut, ventricular pressure _____ but volume and fiber length remain unchanged.

Isovolumetric Relaxation

For a brief period of time (0.02 to 0.06 sec), when all heart values remain shut, ventricular pressure _____ but volume and fiber length remain unchanged.

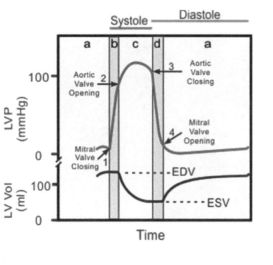
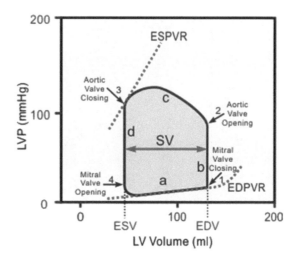

Pipes of the CV System

- **Arteries**
    - thick-walled, high pressure tubing that conducts oxygenated blood
    - Have smooth muscle cells and endothelial cells
- **Arterioles**
    - smaller branched arteries, circular layers of connective tissue
    - Constrict or relax changing the resistance to blood flow
    - Also known as "_____"
- **Capillaries**
    - **Single** layer of **endothelial cells** line capillary wall
    - **NO** smooth muscle
    - Diameter reduced to only allow 1 blood cell at a time
    - Dormant capillaries open during exercise
    - Increased pressure
    - Local metabolites
    - Blood cell takes approximately 1.5 seconds to pass
- **Venules**
    - small veins that collect deoxygenated blood from capillaries
- **Veins**
    - thin-walled, lower pressure
    - Also have smooth muscle cells (but less than arteries) and endothelial cells
- **Capacitance Vessels**
    - act as a blood reservoir, holding _____% of blood volume (can be called upon during exercise)

Structural Make Up

Distribution of Blood at Rest

Heart	=	_____ %
Arteries	=	_____ %
Arterioles, capillaries	=	_____ %
Veins	=	_____ %
Pulmonary system	=	_____ %

Venous System

- **Venous return**
  - Valves within the veins allow blood to flow in only one direction toward the heart
  - The smallest muscular contractions or minor pressure changes within the thoracic cavity with breathing readily compress the veins
  - The alternate compression and relaxation of veins and the one-way action of their valves provide a "milking" action that propels blood back to the heart
  - Without valves, blood would stagnate in veins of the extremities and people would faint every time they stood up because of reduced venous return and cerebral blood flow

- **Venous pooling**
  - May induce fainting from insufficient cerebral blood supply

- **Active "Cool Down"**
  - Moderate exercise in recovery facilitates blood flow to the heart

Varicose Veins

- Veins fail to maintain their one-way blood flow
- Blood gathers in veins and they become excessively distended and painful
- Phlebitis occurs where the venous wall becomes inflamed and progressively deteriorates—vessel removal necessary
- Exercise does not prevent varicose veins but can minimize complications because repeated muscle actions continually propel blood toward the heart

Blood Pressure (BP)

- BP is the _____ exerted by _____ on the walls of *blood vessels*, and is one of the principal *vital signs*.
- During each heartbeat, BP varies between a maximum (*systolic*) and a minimum (*diastolic*) pressure.
- The mean BP decreases as the *circulating blood* moves away from the *heart* through *arteries*, has its greatest decrease in the small arteries and *arterioles*, and continues to decrease as the blood moves through the *capillaries* and back to the heart through *veins*.
- Systolic blood pressure (SBP)
    - Highest arterial pressure measured after left ventricular contraction (systole)
- Diastolic blood pressure (DBP)
    - Lowest arterial pressure measured during left ventricular relaxation (diastole)
- Mean blood pressure (MAP)
    - as the average arterial pressure during a single cardiac cycle
    - Averages 93 mmHg at rest
    - $MAP = DBP + [0.333 (SBP - DBP)]$
    - *MAP* is considered to be the *perfusion pressure* seen by *organs* in the body.
    - *MAP* below 60 mmHg for an appreciable time, the end organ will not get enough blood flow, and will become *ischemic*.

BP Range

BP category	SBP (mmHg)		DBP (mmHg)
Normal	<120	&	<80
Elevated	120–129	&	<80
High BP (Stage 1)	130–139	or	80–89
High BP (Stage 2)	>140	or	>90
Hypertensive Crisis	>180	&/or	>120

Hypertension (HTN)
- Hardened arteries and neural hyperactivity cause increased resistance
- 95% of cases are idiopathic (of unknown etiology)
- Definition ≥ 130/90
- Associated with arteriosclerosis, heart disease, stroke, and kidney failure
- ↓ 2 mmHg ↓ death from stroke by 6% and heart disease by 4%
- BP ↓ prevents stroke and vascular disease and may ↓ the progression of dementia and cognitive impairment

Pressure across the Systemic Circulation

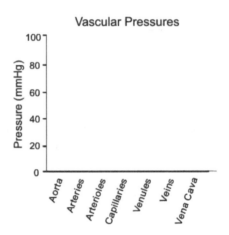

Factors That Influence Arterial BP
- _____ increases
- _____ increases
- _____ increases
- Blood viscosity increases
- Total peripheral resistance (TPR) increases

Total Peripheral Resistance
- The body uses blood vessel diameter to help regulate BP.
- Nerves controlling the muscle fibers can cause the vessel to contract (vasoconstriction) or to expand (vasodilation).
- When BP is too high, blood vessels expand to allow more blood flow. This decreases TPR and lowers BP.
- When BP is low, vessels constrict to increase TPR and BP.

Cardiac Output (CO) Which Includes HR and Stroke Volume (SV)
- CO is the amount of blood pumped by each ventricle per unit of time.
- In a normal person at rest, CO is approximately 5,000 mL/min (5 L/min).

- CO is defined as the amount of blood that is ejected by one ventricle in a one minute period of time.
- CO = MAP/TPR
- TPR = MAP/CO
- At rest:
  - SBP = 126
  - DBP = 80
  - CO = 5.0 L/min
  - TPR = _____

The Role of Exercise on BP, TPR, and CO.

Steady-Rate Exercise

- Vasodilation (active muscles) _____ TPR to _____ blood flow to the peripheral vasculature.
- Muscle contraction and relaxation "milks" blood back to the heart (venous return).
- Increase blood flow during steady-rate exercise rapidly _____ SBP during the first few minutes of exercise.
- As exercise continues, SBP gradually decreases because the arterioles (in active muscles) continue to dilate = decreases TPR.

Graded Exercise

SBP increases rapidly at start of exercise, then SBP increases linearly with exercise intensity

DPB remains stable or decreases slightly

Max SBP may reach 200+mmHg despite reduced TPR

This level of BP most likely reflects the heart's large CO during maximal exercise by individuals with high aerobic capacity

Resistance Exercise

Concentric (shortening) contractions compresses peripheral vasculature causing an increase in TPR

Magnitude of increase in related to the intensity of effort and amount of muscle mass used

CO and TPR during Exercise

- **During exercise:**
  - SBP = 210
  - DBP = 90
  - CO = 20 L/min
  - TPR =

Chapter 9—General Overview of the Cardiovascular System   113

Upper-Body Exercise (UBE) at Max

- **Maximal** exercise
  - $\dot{V}O_2$ values are typically 20 to 30% below those of lower-body exercise (LBE)
  - Lower max HR and pulmonary ventilation
  - Smaller musculature activated

Submax UBE

- UBE requires greater oxygen consumption than LBE at any given submaximal power output
  - Lower mechanical efficiency
  - Recruitment of stabilizing musculature
- UBE provides greater physiological strain than LBE for any given submaximal power output
  - Higher HR, Ve, BP, and RPE

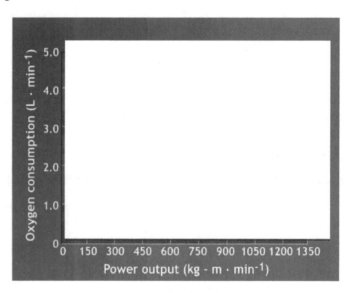

Hypotensive Recovery Response

- *After* a bout of sustained light-to-moderate exercise, _____ temporarily _____ below pre-exercising levels for up to _____ hours in normal and hypertensive subjects.
- Possible explanation:
  - Blood pools in skeletal muscle vascular beds during recovery → decreased central blood volume → decreased atrial filling pressure → lower BP

Exaggerated BP Response during Exercise

- Peak exercise SBP ≥ 210 mmHg for men ≥ 190 mmHg for women
- SBP ≥ 200 mmHg at Exercise Workload of about 6 to 7 METs

What Is the Clinical Significance of a HTN Response?

- Future development of hypertension
- Increased risk for CV mortality and CV events
- Presence of cardiac hypertrophy

HEART'S BLOOD SUPPLY

Coronary Circulation

- **NO** nutrients are taken from the blood flowing to the heart chambers
- Coronary circulation supplies the heart muscle 5% (250 mL) of total output
  - Right and left coronary arteries start at aorta behind aortic valve
  - Arteries divide into a dense capillary network that feeds the myocardium
  - Coronary sinus and anterior cardiac veins collect blood and empty directly into right atrium

Myocardial Oxygen Utilization

- At rest, the myocardium extracts _____% of the oxygen from the blood flowing in the coronary vessels
  - Most other tissues only use approximately _____%
- In vigorous exercise, coronary blood flow increases 4 to 6 times above resting level

Impaired Coronary Blood Supply

- Cardiac muscle purely _____.
- If blood flow is interrupted, chest pain results (angina pectoris)
- Exercise increases energy requirements
  - Stress test = used as a diagnostic tool for myocardial blood flow (ischemia)
- A blood clot within these vessels results in myocardial infarction
  - Damage mild to severe (necrosis = cell death)

Ischemia

- a restriction in blood supply to tissues

Hypoxia

- a region of the body is deprived of adequate O_2 supply

Infarction

- is tissue death (necrosis) caused by a local lack of oxygen

Chapter 9—General Overview of the Cardiovascular System   115

MEASURING MYOCARDIAL WORK

Rate Pressure Product (RPP)

- Provides an noninvasive estimate of myocardial workload (myocardial oxygen uptake)
- RPP = _____ × _____
- RPP = _____ relationship with exercise intensity
- Static exercise: greater increase in SBP than dynamic exercise and therefore a higher myocardial workload (RPP) than dynamic exercise
- Chronic exposure to a higher myocardial workload can lead to cardiac hypertrophy

Cardiac Energy Supply

- Almost exclusively *aerobic energy metabolism*
- Primary source of energy is long-chain fatty acids, glucose, and lactate formed in skeletal muscle
- Prolonged submax exercise = combination of glucose, fatty acids, and lactate
- Maximal exercise = mainly Lactate

CV Regulation and Integration

- Cardiac muscle has an ability to maintain its own rhythm (i.e., heart rate [HR])
- Without extrinsic stimuli, the intrinsic HR is approximately 100 bpm
- Extrinsic control of the heart (i.e., neurohumoral factors) can adjust HR from 40 bpm at rest to 220 bpm at peak exercise

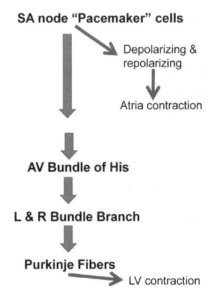

Purkinje system fibers transmit electrical impulses six times faster than normal ventricular muscle fibers.

Electrical delay throughout the heart

- 0.10-second delay allows atria to contract before ventricles (filling)
- 0.06 seconds time till ventricles contract upon stimulation

Electrocardiogram (ECG)

- Records the electrical activity of the heart
- P wave
  - Atrial _____.
- QRS complex
  - Ventricular _____ and atrial _____.
- T wave
  - Ventricular repolarization
- ECG abnormalities may indicate coronary heart disease
  - ST-segment depression can indicate MI

Relationship between Electrical Events and the ECG

Normal ECG

Diagnostic Use of the ECG during Exercise

- Graded exercise test to evaluate cardiac function
  - Observe ECG during exercise
  - Also observe changes in BP
- Atherosclerosis
  - Fatty plaque that narrows coronary arteries
  - Reduces blood flow to myocardium
    - Myocardial ischemia
- ST-segment depression
  - Suggests myocardial ischemia

ST-Segment Depression on the ECG

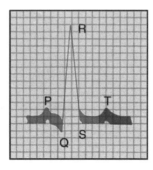 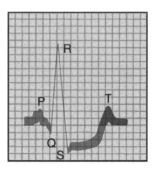

Normal   Ischemia

Obtaining a Rhythm Strip

- Hardwire units: electrodes are placed on the patient and the wires are connected to a cardiac monitor near the patient.
- Telemetry units: electrodes are also placed on the patient, EXCEPT, the wires are connected to a battery-powered transmitter that sends electrical signals to a monitor at another location where the signals are displayed on a monitor screen.

Electrodes

- The area is cleaned with a gauze pad and alcohol to remove any oils from the skin
- Electrodes are place on the skin at specific locations on the torso
- The lead cables are then plugged into a telemetry transmitter or a nearby ECG monitor

Electrode Placement

Right Arm (RA):

- Mid-line and under the right clavicle

Left Arm (LA):

- Mid-line and under the left clavicle

Left Leg (LL):

- In front of the left bicep at the level of the Xiphoid process

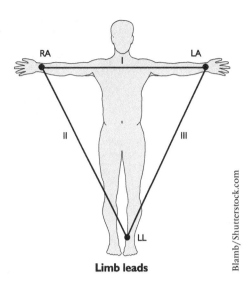

Limb leads

The electrodes for leads I, II, and III are at equidistance from the heart and form a triangle known as Einthoven's triangle

Each side of the triangle is named (Leads I, II, and III) and represents three different views of the heart

Lead I is commonly used to monitor the upper chambers of the heart known as the atria

Lead II looks at the heart from the upper right down to the lower left.

- It is most often known as the "monitoring lead"

Lead III looks at the lateral, left side of the heart and monitors the left ventricle's function of pushing blood out to the rest of the body

Determining TIME and ENERGY

- The lines on the ECG paper are spaced at specific intervals
- Horizontal (left-to-right) markings represent time
- Vertical markings represent voltage or the energy of each signal
- The small horizontal boxes represent 0.04 seconds
- The small vertical boxes represent 0.1mV (millivolts) or 1/1000 of a volt
- Standard paper speed is set at 25 mm/second
- 1 second uses 25 small (horizontal boxes)
- The energy from a single 9 volt battery would take up 90,000 small vertical boxes!

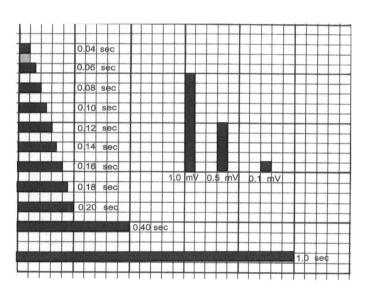

Chapter 9—General Overview of the Cardiovascular System 119

Cardiac and Skeletal Muscle

Similarities

- Both contain _____ and _____ filaments that slide closer together during contraction.

- Both can be electrically excited

- Both show _____ _____ that move along the surface membrane, carrying excitation to all parts of the muscle.

Differences

- The duration of the action potential is 100× longer in cardiac than in skeletal muscle resulting in a long *refractory (rest) period.*

  - The refractory period cancels out any electrical stimulus that occurs before the heart has a chance to rest.

  - Relaxation between the beats is essential to give the heart a chance to fill with blood before the next beat.

  - Cardiac muscle contractions are always brief twitches

- Skeletal muscle contractions resulting from repetitive stimulation can "summate" to cause a smooth and sustained contraction (tetanus).

- Cardiac muscles are interconnected by "gap-junctions" that allow the action potentials to pass from one cell to another to ensure that all of the heart's cells participate in the contraction.

- The entire heart contracts as All-or-None.

- Skeletal muscle will only contract if it receives an electrical impulse.

- Only the fibers connected to that motor neuron will contract.

- Cardiac muscle excites itself

  - Nerves that carry impulses to the heart influence the rate and strength of the contraction, but DO NOT initiate the heartbeat.

  - If the autonomic nerves are destroyed (autonomic neuropathy), the heart continues to beat.

Areas of the Heart That Can Initiate a Rhythm and the Intrinsic Rate

- Sinus node: _____-_____bpm

- Atrial tissue: _____-_____bpm

- Junctional or nodal rhythm (signals from the AV node): _____-_____bpm

- Ventricular tissue _____-_____bpm

Extrinsic HR Regulation

- Functions to accelerate HR in anticipation of exercise, *and* adjust HR as exercise intensity increases or decreases

- Range 20 to 200 bpm (dependent on physical fitness)

- CV control center is located in the medulla and controls HR
- Neural influences superimpose on the inherent rhythm of the myocardium

Sympathetic and Parasympathetic Control

- Sympathetic influence/stimulation
    - _____ medulla portion of adrenal gland
    - Results in tachycardia (SA node and contractility)
- Parasympathetic influence
    - _____ vagal influence
    - Results in bradycardia (slow HR)
- Cortical influence
    - Anticipatory HR

Sympathetic Control on Blood Flow

Mechanism is NE via adrenergic fibers that lie within smooth muscle of small arteries, arterioles, and precapillary sphincters

Inactive Tissue

- Renal, splanchnic, and inactive skeletal muscle
- Produces systemic vasoconstriction of inactive muscle

Active Tissue

- Active muscle
    - Decreased SNS activity produces vasodilation of active muscle
    - Allows blood perfusion

SNS Is Fight or Flight

Increase HR and blood flow to the muscle, but decrease blood flow to GI/kidneys . . . you don't need to digest, you need to run!

Parasympathetic Neural Control

- Heart
    - Acetylcholine
        - _____
        - _____
    - 80% of parasympathetic fibers are carried along Vagus nerve (X)
- Periphery
    - Excitation of iris, gall bladder, and coronary arteries
    - Inhibits gut sphincters, intestines, and skin vasculature
    - During the onset of exercise, HR increases by inhibition of PNS

Chapter 9—General Overview of the Cardiovascular System   121

Neural Response during Exercise

- Anticipatory response

    - Motor cortex sends signal to increase sympathetic and decrease parasympathetic discharge

- Exercise

    - _____

    - _____

- What happens?

    - Increased _____ and _____

    - _____ of active skeletal muscles and heart

    - _____ of skin, gut, spleen etc..

    - Increase in arterial _____ _____

    - Further dilation of muscle vasculature

    - Vasconstriction increases _____ _____

Peripheral Input Control of CV Response

- Initial signal to "drive" CV system comes from higher brain centers

    - Due to centrally-generated motor signals

- Fine-tuned by feedback from:

    - Chemoreceptor

        - sensitive to blood _____, _____, and _____ levels

    - Metaboreflex muscle chemoreceptors

        - Sensitive to muscle metabolites (K^+, lactic acid)

        - Exercise pressor reflex

    - Muscle mechanoreceptors (heart, skin, joints)

        - Sensitive to _____ and _____ of muscular movement

    - Baroreceptors

        - Sensitive to changes in arterial _____

BLOOD DISTRIBUTION

Blood Flow Regulation

- Flow = Pressure × Resistance
- Determining factors for TPR to CO:
  - Physical characteristics of the blood (Viscosity)
  - Size of individual vessels
    - Length of conducting tube
    - Diameter of blood vessel

Poiseuille's Law (quantify blood flow resistance)

- Poiseuille's Law (pwah-zweez)
- Flow = (Pressure gradient × Vessel radius^4) / (Vessel length × Viscosity)
  - Most important = Vessel diameter
  - Vessel length and blood viscosity have less impact
  - Of note vessel radius is _____ related to blood flow
  - Of note viscosity _____ related to blood flow

Exercise and Blood Flow

- Nerves and local metabolites act to dilate arterioles in active muscle beds
- Visceral vasoconstriction and muscle pump bring blood to central circulation

Example:

- Kidneys
  - Rest approximately 1100 mL per minute (approximately 20% of Q)
  - Exercise approximately 250 mL per minute (approximately 1% of Q)

Active Muscle

- Dormant capillaries (1 out of 40 open) at rest
  - Three functions of opening dormant caps*

Chapter 9—General Overview of the Cardiovascular System   123

- Increase to muscle blood flow
- Large blood volume with only minimal increase in blood flow velocity
- Increase the effective surface area for gas and nutrient exchange between blood and muscle fibers
- Local factors—autoregulatory mechanisms
• $\downarrow$pH, $\uparrow$PCO$_2$, $\uparrow$ADP, $\uparrow$Ca^{++}, $\uparrow$temp, hypoxia, nitric oxide (NO)
• Act directly on precap sphincters and smooth muscle bands of small arteries/arterioles to vasodilate
• Reflect elevated tissue metabolism and increased need for oxygen

Exercise and Blood Flow

Draw pie chart

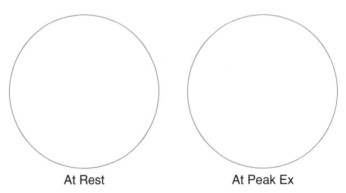

At Rest   At Peak Ex

Mechanism for How NO Regulates Local Blood Flow

Blood Flow to the Heart and Brain

- Heart and brain tissue cannot tolerate a compromised blood supply
- At rest, the myocardium uses approximately _____ % of the oxygen in the blood flowing through the coronary circulation
- During exercise, coronary circulation has a _____ to _____ fold increase
- Cerebral blood flow increases during exercise by approximately 25 to 30% compared with the resting flow

CARDIOVASCULAR DYNAMICS

CO = measure of the functional capacity of the circulatory system to meet the demands for exercise:

$$CO = HR \times SV$$

The relationship between V_{O_2}, CO and the difference between the O_2 content of arterial and mixed venous blood (a–vO_2 diff) embodies the Fick principle:

$$CO = VO_2/\text{a–}vO_2 \text{ diff}$$

Measuring CO Noninvasively

CO_2 rebreathing

$$CO = VCO_2/(\text{v–a } CO_2 \text{ difference}) \times 100$$

Collier Method

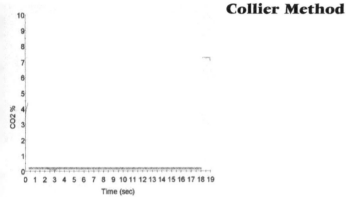

Defares Method

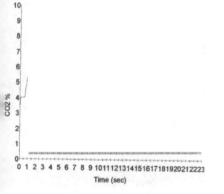

One limitation = requires steady-state exercise – restricting its use to submax exercise.

CO at Rest

		Q (l.min⁻¹)	HR (bpm)	SV (ml)
Rest	Untrained			
	Trained			

Hemodynamics during Exercise

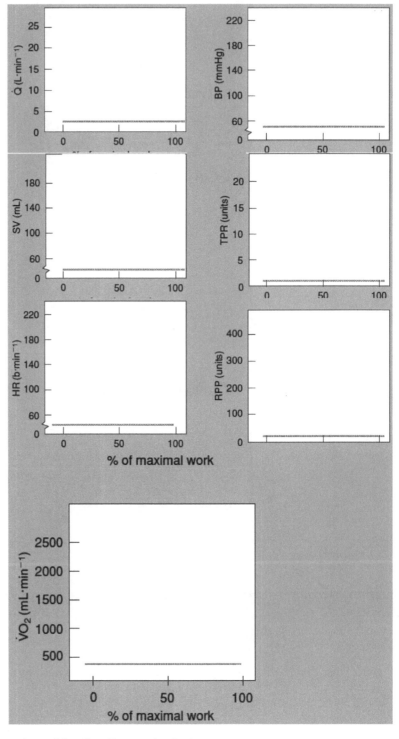

CO at Maximal Exercise

		Q (l.min^{-1})	HR (bpm)	SV (ml)
Rest	Untrained			
	Trained			
Max Ex	Untrained			
	Trained			

The Fick Principle

	VO$_{2max}$ (l.min^{-1})	Q$_{max}$ (l.min^{-1})	HR$_{max}$ (bpm)	SV$_{max}$ (ml)	a-vO$_2$ diff (ml 100 min^{-1})
Untrained					
Trained					
MS					

Aging, Training, and Vo$_{2max}$

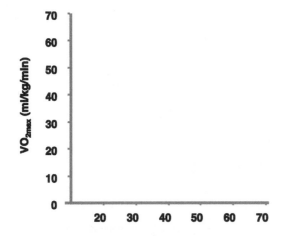

Adaptation to Endurance Training

- **Athletes have greater SV due to:**
  - Increased compliance of the left ventricle, or reduced cardiac stiffness, allows for greater volume during filling
  - Possibly greater contractile state
  - Expanded blood volume
  - Enhanced redistribution of blood volume

SV and Body Position

- **Horizontal**

  Resting SV remains near max, small increase with exercise

  - Upright

  Decreased preload relative to horizontal position

  - Gravity counters the return flow of blood to the heart

  SV increases to approach supine max with intensity

Starling Law of the Heart

- An increase in end-diastolic volume (increased preload) stretches myocardial fibers, causing a powerful ejection stroke as the heart contracts
- Improved contractility of a stretched muscle (within a limited range) probably relates to a more optimum arrangement of intracellular myofilaments as the muscle stretches

Greater Systolic Emptying

Physiologic mechanisms to increase SV during exercise:

- Enhanced cardiac fill (increase EDV) and contraction (increase ESV)
  - Frank–Starling mechanism
  - At rest, approximately 40% of EDV remains in LV
    - Ejection fraction = % ejected per beat
- Increased forceful ejection
  - Via neurohormonal influences

CV Drift

- Alteration to SV and HR during prolonged exercise
- Exercise duration of >15 min
  - Fluid loss
    - Sweating
    - Fluid shift (plasma to tissue)

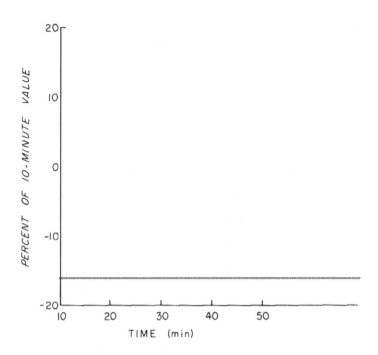

Regulation of CO

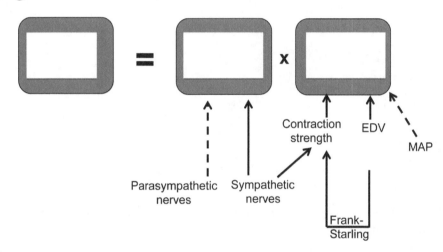

Oxygen Transport

Rearranging Fick equation:

$$Q\ (L/min) = V_{O_2}\ (mL/min)\ /\ \text{a-v}\ O_2\ \text{difference}\ (mL/L)$$

$$V_{O_2}\ (mL/min) = Q\ (L/min) \times \text{a-v}\ O_2\ \text{difference}\ (mL/L)$$

- Oxygen carrying capacity of blood is 20 mL of oxygen per 100 mL of blood or 200 mL/L of blood

CO and Oxygen Transport

- **Rest**
  - 200 mL O_2 per L of blood
  - If CO = 5L then, (5 × 200) 1000 mL of oxygen available
  - Resting oxygen consumption (250 mL)
  - 750 mL returns = oxygen reserve

- **Max exercise**
  - CO increases to 20 to 22 L/min at max effort
  - 4400 mL O_2 available (22 × 200)
  - If increase SV (with training)
  - (35 × 200) 7000 mL O_2

Max CO and VO_{2max}

- Direct association for sedentary and endurance-trained athletes
- 6:1 ratio increase in CO with each liter increase in Vo_2max
- Training:
  - Proportionate increase in CO_{max} accompanies increases in Vo_2max

OXYGEN TRANSPORT

- Athletes can experience a 20-fold increase in Vo_2 from rest to max
- If only achieved by flow, Q would need to increase from 5L/min to 100L/min (5 × 20)
- This large increase is not needed due to large reserve of oxygen available
- Arterial O_2 =200 mL/L
- Venous O_2 =150 mL/L
- Only 25% is being extracted at rest

Oxygen Extraction

- The increase in Vo_2 is achieved by both increased CO and an expanded a–vO_2
- Image shows a progressive expansion of the a–vO_2 difference from rest to max exercise

Draw a-vo$_2$ Figure

Exercise: Factors Affecting a-v O_2

- Diverted more blood to active muscles
- Increased capillary density "enlarges the interface" for nutrient and metabolic gas exchange
    - Large capillary to fiber ratio in individuals exhibiting large a-v O_2 differences during exercise
- Increased size and number of mitochondria and aerobic enzymes (i.e., citrate synthase) improve ATP production aerobically
- Enhanced release of O_2 by hemoglobin

Determinants of Vo_{2max}

Peripheral Factors

- Muscle blood flow
- Capillary density
- O_2 Diffusion
- O_2 extraction
- Hb–O_2 affinity
- Muscle fiber profiles

Central Factors

- CO
- Arterial pressure
- Hemoglobin
- Ventilation
- O_2 diffusion
- Hb–O_2 affinity
- Alveolar VE perfusion ratio

Factors Affecting Vo_{2max}

Intrinsic

- Genetic
- Gender
- Body composition
- Muscle mass
- Age
- Pathologies

Extrinsic

- Activity levels
- Time of day

- Sleep deprivation
- Dietary intake
- Nutritional status
- Environment

Clinical Importance of Exercise

- Exercise prescription
    - A standard submaximal exercise load with the upper body produces greater metabolic and physiologic strain than leg exercise
    - Exercise Rx based on running/biking do not apply to arm exercise
    - Low correlations between arm and leg exercise VO_2

Physical Inactivity

Effect of bed rest on VO_{2max}

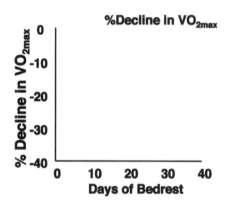

Data from VA Convertino MSSE 1997

Physical Inactivity/Detraining

Review Questions: Chapter 9: Part One

(For true and false questions that are false, indicate what would make the question true)

1. At rest, the greatest percentage of blood volume will be located in the

    a. heart.

    b. lungs.

    c. aorta and arteries.

    d. veins.

    e. capillaries.

2.3.4. (Circle correct choice of bold terms.) **Oxygenated/deoxygenated** blood passes through the **tricuspid/mitral** valve to the left ventricle where the blood is pumped through the **pulmonary/aortic** valve.

5. *True or False*:

    Arteries carry only oxygenated blood and veins carry only deoxygenated blood.

Matching:

6. High-pressure, thick-walled vessels _____

7. Low-pressure, thin-walled vessels _____

8. Single endothelial cells line wall of vessel _____

9. Collect deoxygenated blood from capillaries _____

    a. Capillaries

    b. Arteries

    c. Veins

    d. Venules

10. What is the purpose of "cooling down" after exercise?

11. The vessels that have the highest pressure to lowest pressure in order are:

    a. arteries, arterioles, venules, capillaries, veins.

    b. arteries, arterioles, capillaries, venules, veins.

    c. arteries, arterioles, venules, veins, capillaries.

    d. arteries, arterioles, capillaries, veins, venules.

12. The vessels that have the highest velocity to lowest velocity in order are

    a. arteries, veins, capillaries.

    b. arteries, capillaries, veins.

    c. veins, capillaries, arteries.

    d. none of the above.

Chapters 9—General Overview of the Cardiovascular System   133

Matching:

13. Cardiac output (CO) _____

14. Total peripheral resistance (TPR) _____

15. Blood pressure _____

16. Systolic blood pressure _____

17. Diastolic blood pressure _____

    a. (Cardiac output) × (total peripheral resistance)

    b. Pressure during ventricular relaxation

    c. (Heart rate) × (stroke volume)

    d. Sum of resistance in all peripheral vessels

    e. Pressure during ventricular contraction

18. What is the mean arterial pressure of a person with a blood pressure of 142/94?

19. Hypertension is caused primarily by

    a. smoking.

    b. kidney disease.

    c. alcoholism.

    d. none of the above; most cases of hypertension are idiopathic.

20. *True or False:*

In general, blood pressure increases more during resistance exercise than during aerobic exercise.

21. *True or False:*

In response to exercise, systolic blood pressure and diastolic blood pressure will rise. (Explain your answer.)

22. (Circle correct choice of bold terms.) The pulmonary artery carries **oxygenated/deoxygenated** blood.

23. As blood flows through the heart's chambers:

    a. nutrients are taken from the blood, which supports the heart.

    b. no nutrients are taken from the blood.

24. The coronary circulation supplies the _____ muscle.

25. (Circle correct choice of bold terms.) The greatest amount of blood flow to the heart occurs during **systole/diastole**.

26. Trace an RBC throughout the main parts of the cardiovascular system, starting and ending in the right atrium.

27. Graph the relationship between systolic, diastolic, and mean arterial pressure to increased work (show the results you would expect during a graded exercise test to maximum).

28. a. (Circle correct choice of bold terms.) Blood pressure may **fall/ rise** following a bout of submaximal exercise.

    b. Explain the mechanism(s) for this affect.

29. a. (Circle correct choice of bold terms.) Blood pressure is **higher/ lower** in the arms versus the legs when exercising each at the a given percentage of VO2 max.

    b. Explain the mechanism(s) for this affect.

30. a. The rate-pressure product is determined by:

    b. How is this measure related to angina?

Review Questions: Chapter 9: Part Two

(For true and false questions that are false, indicate what would make the question true)

1. The _____, _____, _____, and _____ are structures within the heart that regulate its rate. (Answer must be in order of activation.)

2. *True or False:*

   The AV node is also known as the pacemaker of the heart.

3. The P-wave represents the _____ of the _____.

   a. repolarization; atria

   b. repolarization; ventricles

   c. depolarization; atria

   d. depolarization; ventricles

Matching:

4. Ventricular depolarization and repolarization _____

5. Ventricular depolarization _____

6. Atrial depolarization _____

7. Electrical transmission from the atria to the ventricle _____

8. Atrial repolarization _____

9. Ventricular repolarization _____

10. Part of an ECG that is an indicator of myocardial oxygen demand and supply _____

    a. P-wave

    b. P-R interval

    c. QRS complex

    d. T-wave

    e. S-T segment

    f. Q-T interval

11. Where is the cardiovascular control center located?

12. An inotropic effect, by definition, causes greater _____.

13. An increase in epinephrine and norepinephrine will cause _____, which is a heart rate _____ than _____ beats per minute.

    a. tachycardia; more; 60

    b. tachycardia; more; 100

    c. bradycardia; less; 60

    d. bradycardia; more; 100

14. Eighty percent of parasympathetic nerve fibers are carried along the _____ nerve.

Chapters 9—General Overview of the Cardiovascular System   137

15. *True or False:*

    Acetylcholine has no effect on myocardial contractility.

16. Which of the following is a response to exercise?

    I. Increase in heart rate

    II. Vasodilation of vessels in active muscle and heart

    III. Vasoconstriction causing decreased venous return

    IV. Increase in arterial blood pressure

    V. Vasodilation of vessels of skin and gut

    VI. Decrease in sympathetic and increase in parasympathetic discharge

    a. I, II ,III , IV

    b. I, II, III, IV, V

    c. I, II, IV

    d. I, II, IV, VI

    e. I, II, IV, V

17. Baroreceptors located in the aortic arch and carotid sinus function to inhibit _____ output and prevent a significant increase in _____.

    a. parasympathetic; heart rate

    b. parasympathetic; blood pressure

    c. sympathetic; heart rate

    d. sympathetic; blood pressure

18. *True or False:*

    The baroreceptor reflex is overridden during exercise.

19. An intern in the Human Performance Laboratory decides to take a client's heart rate by pressing and applying pressure to the carotid artery. What will most likely happen to this client if enough pressure is applied?

    a. The client's heart rate will increase.

    b. The client's heart rate will decrease.

    c. The client's heart rate will not change.

20. According to Poiseuille's Law, which factor has the largest impact on blood flow?

    a. blood viscosity

    b. vessel length

    c. vessel radius or diameter

    d. pressure gradient

    e. none of the above

138   Chapters 9—General Overview of the Cardiovascular System

21. During exercise, which two factors help bring blood back to the central circulation (heart)?

22. Compared to at rest, during heavy exercise blood flow increases significantly in which system(s)?

    a. Digestive system

    b. Kidneys

    c. Heart

    d. Brain

    e. Bone

    f. Skeletal muscle

23. Compared to at rest, during heavy exercise blood flow decreases significantly in which system(s)?

    a. Digestive system

    b. Kidneys

    c. Heart

    d. Brain

    e. Skeletal muscle

24. Discuss the reason why blood flow needs to be increased/decreased to the following tissues during strenuous exercise (include the mechanisms of how this is achieved).

    a. Kidney

    b. Heart muscle

25. *True or False:*

    Endothelial cells within blood vessels release nitric oxide, resulting in vasodilation of the vessel.

26. Briefly discuss the primary difference in the heart-rate response to a maximal graded exercise test for a person who has undergone a heart transplant as compared with an individual with a normal, healthy heart. What causes this difference?

27. Draw and label each part of a normal ECG.

28. The _____ represents recovery of the Purkinje or ventricular conduction fibers.

29. Sinus _____ is a heart rate greater than 100 beats per minute.

30. On an ECG recording, if the R-R interval is separated by two large boxes, the heart rate would be _____.

Chapters 9—General Overview of the Cardiovascular System   139

Review Questions: Chapter 9: Part Three

(For true and false questions that are false, indicate what would make the question true)

1. Cardiac output is defined as the _____ multiplied by the _____.

2. What letter stands for cardiac output?

3. What is the stroke volume of a woman with a resting heart rate of 65 beats per minute?

4. Resting heart rate _____ with endurance training due to a(n) _____ in sympathetic output and a(n) _____ in parasympathetic output.

    a. increases; increase; decrease

    b. increases; increase; increase

    c. decreases; increase; decrease

    d. decreases; decrease; increase

5. Although endurance training decreases resting heart rate, cardiac output remains unchanged from that of an untrained person. How is this possible?

6. A client in the HPL is exercising at a light to moderate intensity. After some time, the client decides to increase the intensity by exercising vigorously. How will cardiac output increase when the client is exercising vigorously?

    a. Both heart rate and stroke volume will increase the cardiac output.

    b. Only stroke volume will increase the cardiac output.

    c. Only heart rate will increase the cardiac output.

7. How is stroke volume increased during exercise?

8. End-diastolic volume is defined as the volume of blood in the

    a. atria after relaxation

    b. atria after contraction

    c. ventricle after the ventricle contracts

    d. ventricle at the end of filling (diastole)

9. At rest, the ejection fraction is approximately:

    a. 40%.

    b. 60%.

    c. 80%.

10. *True or False:*

    There is a relationship between cardiac output and maximal oxygen consumption (VO_2 max).

11. For every liter increase in a person's VO_2 max, there is an increase in cardiac output of _____ L/min.

Chapters 9—General Overview of the Cardiovascular System   141

12. (Circle the correct choice of bold terms.) Upper-body exercises require a higher/lower oxygen consumption at a given submaximal power output.

13. By using the direct Fick method, cardiac output can be measured. What information would be needed?

   a. average difference between O_2 content in arterial and mixed venous blood

   b. O_2 consumption during 1 min

   c. both a and b

   d. none of the above

14. What are the units for cardiac output (hint: look at the CO equation)?

15. What are the average values of cardiac output (in L) for a male and female, respectively?

   a. 8, 7

   b. 5, 4

   c. 7, 6

   d. 4, 3

16. *True or False:*

   Ejection fraction is increased by increasing preload.

17. (Circle the correct choice of bold terms.) Increased/Decreased compliance of the heart allows for an increased end-diastolic volume.

18. *True or False:*

   Beta blockers will prevent significant increases in heart rate during exercise.

19. Define *cardiovascular drift*. Briefly discuss how this may occur when exercising in a hot, humid environment.

20. a. Maximal VO_2 is determined by maximal _____ and _____ .

   b. Briefly discuss how exercise training affects both.

Chapters 9

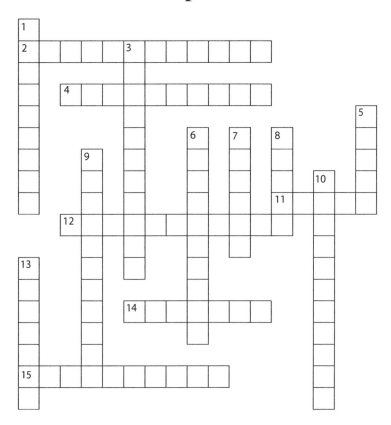

ACROSS

2 Abnormally high blood pressure.
4 Signal selectrical changes from ventricular depolarization on an ECG.
11 Represents ventricular repolarization on an ECG.
12 Describes reduced heart rate.
14 Small veins.
15 Small arterial branches.

DOWN

1 Inflamed venous wall which progressively deteriorates.
3 Describes heart rate acceleration.
5 Represents depolarization of the atria on an ECG.
6 The heart muscle.
7 Pacemaker of the heart.
8 Blood is pumped from the left ventricle.
9 Relaxing factor that facilitates blood vessel dilation and decreases vascular resistance.
10 Microscopically small blood vessels.
13 The stretch of the ventricles in diastole to produce a more forceful ejection stroke.

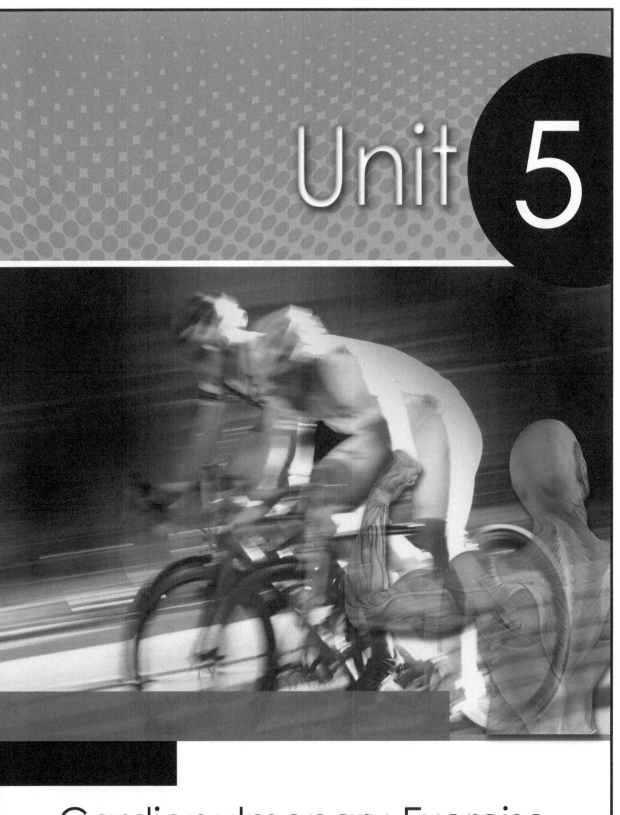

Unit 5

Cardiopulmonary Exercise Physiology

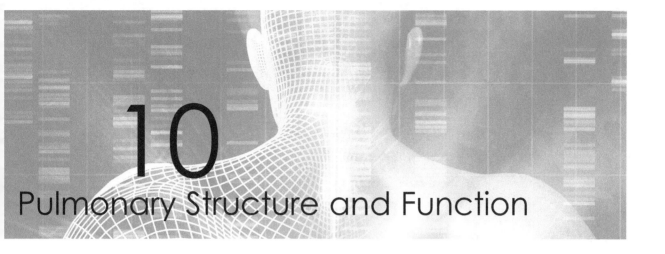

10
Pulmonary Structure and Function

STRUCTURE AND FUNCTION OF THE LUNG:

Is fragile and delicate (but also strong).

Is the only organ (other than the heart) to receive the entire cardiac output.

Functions of lung include:

- Gas exchange !!!
- Filtering (blood and air)
  - Captures inhaled particles
  - Breakdown vasoactive substances
    - Converts angiotensin I to angiotensin II (angiotensin converting enzyme [ACE] is in the lungs)
    - Bradykinin (80% inactivated in lung)
    - Serotonin (almost completely removed)
    - Norepinephrine (up to 30% removed)
    - PGE2 and PGF2 alpha (almost completely removed)
    - Leukotrienes (almost completely removed)
- Vocalizations (speaking, singing, etc.)

Lung Dynamics:

At Rest:

O_2 consumed (VO_2) approximately 250 mL/min

CO_2 produced (VCO_2) approximately 300 mL/min

Ventilation approximately 5,000 mL/min (5 L/min)

Exercise:

V_{O_2} approximately 3,000 mL/min (up to 6,250 mL/min in athletes)

V_{CO_2} approximately 3,000 mL/min (up to 7,000 mL/min in athletes)

Ventilation > 60,000 mL/min (60 L/min)

Anatomy of the Lung:

a. Upper airways

b. Airways (lung)

- Trachea
- Bronchi
- Bronchioles
- Alveoli

c. Lung

- Lobes
- Pleural space

d. Muscles

- Diaphragm
- Intercostals

e. Alveoli:

   i. The lungs contain between 300 and 600 million air sacs called alveoli

   ii. Thin walled (single epithelial cell)

   iii. Elastic

   iv. Pores of Kohn allow for even dispersion of surfactant

   v. Surfactant decreases surface tension

   vi. Pores also allow for gas interchange between alveoli

   vii. Provide a large surface area (50 to 100 m^2) for gas exchange

   viii. Transfer of gas across the lung occurs via *diffusion*!

      a. Fick's Law of Diffusion (explains gas exchange across the alveolar membrane)

$$\dot{V}_{gas} \propto \frac{A}{T} \cdot D \cdot (P_1 - P_2)$$

   ix. Surfactant

- Resistance to expansion of the lungs increases during inspiration due to surface tension on alveoli.

148   Chapter 10—Pulmonary Structure and Function

- Surfactant:a lipoprotein mix of phospholipids, proteins, and Ca^{2+} produced by alveolar epithelial cells—mixes with fluid around alveoli.

- Surfactant disrupts and lowers surface tension (Surface tension is force acting only at a gas-liquid interface).

- Law of Laplace shows that

$$Pressure\ (P) = \frac{4 \times Surface\ Tension\ (T)}{Radius\ (r)}$$

Lungs are highly vascularized to allow for gas exchange:

- Receives the entire cardiac output

- Red blood cell (RBC) transit time in lung capillaries is approximately 0.75 seconds (approximately 0.25 seconds with exercise)

Mechanics of Ventilation:

- Inspiration—air moves into the lungs

  - At rest, the diaphragm contracts and moves down approximately 10 cm

  - Chest cavity elongates and enlarges and air expands in lungs

  - Intrapulmonary pressure decreases

    - Air moves into the lung due to the **Universal Gas Law (PV = nRT)**, when simplified this expressed as **PV = T**.

    - If temperature is constant, *pressure and volume are inversely related* (known as **Boyles Law**) $\uparrow$**P** $\downarrow$**V = k**

  - Air is forced into the lungs until $P_I = P_A$

- Expiration—air moves to the atmosphere

  - At rest and during light exercise, respiratory muscles are normally *passive*

    - Inspiratory muscles relax

    - Lung is elastic (stretched lung tissue recoils)

  - During heavy exercise respiratory muscle at *active*

    - Internal intercostals

    - Abdominal muscles assist

Lung Volumes and Capacities

Normal lung volumes depend on:

- Age

- Sex

- Stature (i.e. height)

- Race

Chapter 10—Pulmonary Structure and Function   149

Draw an example of flow volume obtained from a spirometer that is used to measure lung's basic lung volumes. **Label the axes appropriately with the appropriate units.**

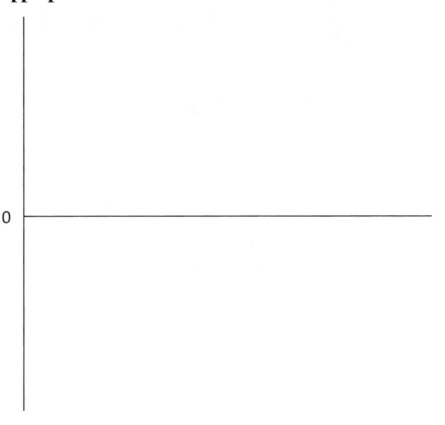

Static Lung Volumes

- TV (tidal volume)   0.4–1.0 L air/breath
- IRV (inspiratory reserve volume)   2.5–3.5 L
- ERV (expiratory reserve volume)   1.0–1.5 L
- VC (vital capacity)   3.0–5.0 L
- RV (residual volume)   0.8–1.4 L

Helium dilution technique: used to measure lung volumes that cannot be measured by basic spirometry.

$$V_1 \times C_1 = V_2 \times C_2$$

During exercise,

- IRV and ERV decrease, as TV increases
- Both the rate and depth of breathing increase.
- Increases in TV depth become limited as ventilation increases (for example during heavy exercise), leaving only respiratory rate to increase ventilation further.

Dynamic Lung Volumes:

- Forced vital capacity (FVC) plotted against time or velocity of flow
- Forced expired volume (FEV) at 1 second = FEV_1

- Velocity of flow is influenced by lung compliance (stiffness of the lung)

$$\text{Compliance}_{\text{LUNG}} = \Delta\text{Volume}/\Delta\text{Pressure}$$

- FEV_1/FVC indicates pulmonary airflow characteristics
  - Healthy people average approximately 80 to 85% of FVC in 1 second.
  - Obstructive diseases result in significantly lower FEV_1/FVC

Measuring Ventilation:

- **Minute Ventilation ($\dot{V}E$, L/min):** Volume of air moved into or out of the lung each minute.
  - a. Total volume of air breathed each minute

  Tidal volume (TV) $\times$ respiratory frequency (f) = minute ventilation ($\dot{V}E$)

  $$TV \times f = \dot{V}E$$

  $$500 \text{ ml} \times 12 \text{ bpm} = \mathbf{6,000 \text{ mL/min} (6 \text{ L/min})}$$

  - b. Minute ventilation increases dramatically during exercise.

  60 to 120 L/min common, values up to 200 L/min have been reported.

  - c. Despite huge $\dot{V}E$, TV rarely exceed 60% VC.

- **Alveolar Ventilation ($\dot{V}A$: L/min):** Volume of air that reaches the respiratory zone.

  $\dot{V}A$ excludes *anatomic* dead space, therefore

  $$(TV - \text{deadspace}) \times f = \dot{V}A$$

  $$(500 - 150 \text{ mL}) \times 12 = \mathbf{4,200 \text{ mL/min} (4.2 \text{ L/min})}$$

Physiologic Dead Space:

- Occurs in the *respiratory zone* where there should be gas exchange.
- Physiologic dead space is the result of **inadequate blood flow to alveolar lung units**.

Write the **alveolar ventilation equation** (below) and understand what this is telling you!

Hyperventilation:

- An *increase* in alveolar ventilation that exceeds needs of metabolism
- Hyperventilation *decreases* P_{CO_2}.

Hypoventilation:

- A *decrease* in alveolar ventilation that is below needs of metabolism
- Hypoventilation *increases* P_{CO_2}.

Dyspnea:

- Subjective distress in breathing, often described as "shortness of breath"
- During exercise, respiratory muscles may fatigue, resulting in shallow, ineffective breathing, and increased dyspnea.

Maximum Voluntary Ventilation (MVV):

- Provides assessment of entire respiratory system
  - Muscle strength, lung, and chest compliance; airway resistance; and ventilatory control mechanisms
- MVV evaluates ventilatory capacity with rapid and deep breathing for 15 seconds.
  - MVV (L/min) = 15 second volume × 4
  - Average 150 to 200 L/min for young healthy men, slightly lower for female
  - Maneuver is effort dependent!
- MVV in healthy individuals averages 25% > ventilation than occurs during maximum exercise

Valsalva Maneuver:

Closing the glottis following a full inspiration while maximally activating the expiratory muscles.

Physiological consequences:

a. An acute drop in BP may result from a prolonged Valsalva maneuver (*due to effects of increased intrathoracic pressure*)

  - Decreased venous return
  - Decreased flow to brain

b. Dizziness or fainting result

Lung Function, Aerobic Fitness, and Exercise Performance

- Lungs are generally considered to be "over-built". In most healthy individuals the lungs do not limit exercise performance. During maximum exercise the lung is generally not limited by ventilation in most people.
- Little relationship exists among diverse lung volumes and capacities and exercise performance.

Respiratory Tract during Cold-Weather Exercise

- Cold ambient air is warmed as it passes through the conducting zone
- Moisture is lost if the air is cold and dry
- Contributes to
  - Dehydration
  - Dry mouth
  - Irritation of respiratory passages

Review Questions: Chapter 10

(For true and false questions that are false, indicate what would make the question true)

1. Each of the following occur in the lungs *except*:

   a. Gas exchange

   b. Conversion of angiotensin I to angiotensin II

   c. Removal of inhaled particles

   d. Removal of hormones and other vasoactive substances (i.e., norepinephrine, bradykinin, PGE2, etc.)

   e. Extrapulmonary shunting

2. Briefly define the primary purpose of each of the following:

   a. Trachea

   b. Bronchi

   c. Bronchioles

   d. Alveoli

3. The functional unit of the lung is the _____

4. _____ is a lipoprotein mix of phospholipids, proteins, and Ca^{2+} produced by alveolar epithelial cells which disrupts and lowers surface tension of the lung.

5. **True** or **False**: The lungs receive approximately 75% of the cardiac output with each heart beat.

6. List the range of volumes (L of air per breath) for each of the follow static lung volumes:

   a. TV (tidal volume)

   b. IRV (insp. reserve volume)

   c. ERV (exp. reserve volume)

   d. VC (vital capacity)

   e. RV (residual volume)

7. **True** or **False**: During heavy exercise, TV increases considerably more than breathing rate (percentage of resting values).

8. Each of the following are true statements *except*:

   a. Lung volumes vary with age

   b. The size of one's lung can increase with aerobic training.

   c. Women have smaller lungs than men.

   d. Highly fit women tend to have reduced arterial blood O_2 levels during exercise compared to men.

9. Minute ventilation is determined by _____ × _____. What is the normal resting value and maximal exercise values?

Chapter 10—Pulmonary Structure and Function   155

10. Define the following:

    a. Physiological dead space:

    b. Anatomical dead space:

    c. Alveolar ventilation:

11. **True** or **False**: Hyperventilation is an *increase* in alveolar ventilation that *exceeds* needs of metabolism.

12. **True** or **False**: Dyspnea is another name for *hyperventilation*

13. **True** or **False**: Maximal lung capacity often is the limiting factor in maximal aerobic exercise performance.

14. The Valsalva maneuver:

    a. Is a full maximal exhalation against a closed glottis.

    b. Produces an increase in intrathoracic pressure

    c. Results in a significant rise in blood pressure and blood flow to the brain.

    d. a and b

    e. All of these

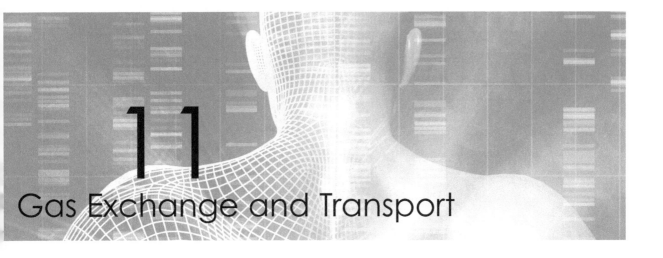

Gas Exchange and Transport

Terminology and Abbreviations:

Primary
V = volume
$\dot{V}$ = volume / time (gas)
P = partial pressure
F = fraction
C = content
S = saturation
$\dot{Q}$ = Blood flow (vol/time)

Secondary
I = inspired
E = expired
A = alveolar
a = arterial
v = venous
$\bar{v}$ = mixed venous (Pulmonary Artery)
T (or lowercase t) = tidal
D (or lowercase d) = dead space

For example: **$\dot{V}E$, $\dot{V}A$, $\dot{V}O_2$, $\dot{V}CO_2$, PAO_2, PaO_2, PvO_2, SaO_2, FIO_2**

O_2 and CO_2 transport, Acid/Base Regulation:

Concentration and partial pressure of respired gases:
- Partial pressure of any gas is equal to the total pressure of a gas times the percentage of concentration of specific gas

Atmospheric Air is principally comprised of oxygen and nitrogen (*fill in the relative % for each gas below*).

O_2 = _____%
CO_2 = _____%
N_2 = _____%

Dalton's Law

Total pressure = Sum of partial pressure of all gases in a mixture

Chapter 11—Gas Exchange and Transport   157

In Ambient Air at Sea level

$PB\ (760\ mmHg) = P_{O_2} + P_{CO_2} + P_{N_2}$

Problem to Solve: *If barometric pressure is 760 mmHg, calculate the partial pressure for*

O_2	= 20.93%	= _____ mmHg, P_{O_2}
CO_2	= 0.03%	= _____ mmHg, P_{CO_2}
N_2	= 79.04%	= _____ mmHg, P_{N_2}

Sum of partial of pressures = 100% = _____ mmHg

In the trachea (air is humidified), therefore water vapor is present and must also be account for:

$PB\ (760\ mmHg) = P_{O_2} + P_{CO_2} + P_{N_2} + P_{H_2O}$

O_2	=	= 149 mmHg, P_{O_2}
CO_2	=	= 0.23 mmHg, P_{CO_2}
N_2	=	= 563 mmHg, P_{N_2}
H_2O at 37 °C	=	= 47 mmHg, P_{H_2O}

Sum of partial of pressures = 100% = **760 mmHg**

In the alveoli of the lung, water vapor and significantly more CO_2 is present, therefore...

$PB\ (760\ mmHg) = P_{O_2} + P_{CO_2} + P_{N_2} + P_{H_2O}$

O_2	= 14–15%	= 100–106 mmHg, P_{O_2}
CO_2	= 5–6%	= 36–43 mmHg, P_{CO_2}
N_2	= 79.04%	= 564 mmHg, P_{N_2}
H_2O at 37 °C	=	= 47 mmHg, P_{H_2O}

Sum of partial of pressures = 100% = **760 mmHg**

Movement of Gas in Air and Fluids Occurs via Diffusion

- Henry's law

  - Gases diffuse from high pressure to low pressure.

- Diffusion rate depends upon

  - Pressure differential

  - Solubility of the gas in the fluid

    i. Solubility:

       CO_2 is about 22 to 25 times more soluble than O_2.

       $CO_2 = 0.067\ mL\ CO_2/mmHg/100\ mL\ blood$

       $O_2 = 0.003\ mL\ O_2/mmHg/100\ mL\ blood$

Gas Exchange in Lungs and Tissues

Exchange of gases between lungs and blood, and gas movement at the tissue level progress **passively by *diffusion* and is dependent on the pressure difference gradient**.

Fick's Law of Diffusion

$$\dot{V}gas \propto \frac{A}{T} \cdot D \cdot (P_1 - P_2)$$

Problem to Solve: Define each component of this equation,

$\dot{V} =$

$A =$

$T =$

$D =$

$P_1 =$

$P_2 =$

Transport of O_2 in the Blood:

Two mechanisms exist for O_2 transport

1. Dissolved in plasma (P_{O_2})

   - O_2 solubility = 0.003 mL O_2/mmHg/100 mL blood
   - That means for each 1 mmHg increase, 0.003 mL O_2 dissolves into plasma.
   - Normal PaO_2 is 100 mmHg, that means
     - 0.3 mL O_2/100 mL blood (or 3 mL O_2/L blood).
   - Dissolved O_2 establishes the P_{O_2} of the blood

2. Bound to Hemoglobin

   - Each of four iron atoms associated with hemoglobin combines with one O_2 molecule.
   - Each gram of Hb combines with 1.34 mL O_2.
   - With normal Hb levels, each dL (100 mL) of blood contains about 20 mL O_2.
   - With 5 L total blood volume = 1000 mL O_2 in blood.

Adding the two separate components yields the total O_2 content in arterial blood (CaO_2)....

Dissolved → 100 × 0.003 = 0.3 mL O_2/dL

+ Bound Hb → 1.34 × 15 × 0.98 = 19.7 mL O_2/dL

= Total O_2 content in arterial blood = 20.0 mL O_2/dL

Draw the O_2 dissociation curve (**make sure to label each axis appropriately**, and indicate where **arterial** and **venous blood** are found on the curve)

Anemia Affects Oxygen Transport:

- Iron deficiency anemia reduces O_2 carrying capacity considerably

- Anything that reduces Hb binding to oxygen reduces O_2 transport

Problem to Solve: If Hb is 5 g/dL and saturation is 50% and PaO_2 is 100 mmHg, calculate the total arterial O_2 content (CaO_2). Show your work!

$$CaO_2 \text{ (mL } O_2/dL) =$$

Arteriovenous O_2 (a–vO_2) Difference

The a–vO_2 difference shows the amount of O_2 extracted by tissues.

For example: If arterial blood contains 20 mL O_2/dL and venous contains 15 mL O_2/dL, then the tissues have extracted (20–15) 5 mL O_2/dL blood.

Bohr Effect

States that hemoglobin's oxygen binding affinity is inversely related to concentration of carbon dioxide and blood acidity.

Question: What does exercise do to the oxygen dissociation curve?

2,3-Diphosphoglycerate (DPG)

- RBCs contain no mitochondria (they must rely on glycolysis for energy)
- 2,3-DPG is a by-product of glycolysis
- 2,3-DPG increases with intense exercise and may increase due to training.
- 2,3-DPG helps deliver O_2 to tissues

Myoglobin, the Muscle's O_2 Store

- Myoglobin is an iron-containing globular protein in skeletal and cardiac muscle
- Stores O_2 intramuscularly
- Myoglobin contains only 1 iron atom
- O_2 is released at low P_{O_2}

Transport of CO_2 in the Blood:

Three mechanisms exist for CO_2 transport

1. Dissolved in plasma (P_{CO_2})

    - approximately 5% CO_2 is transported as dissolved CO_2
    - the dissolved CO_2 establishes the P_{CO_2} of the blood

2. CO_2 transport as carbamino compounds

    - CO_2 reacts directly with amino acids to form carbamino compounds (i.e. Hb, albumin, etc.)
    - Haldane effect: Hb interaction with O_2 reduces its ability to combine with CO_2.
    - This aids in releasing CO_2 in the lungs.

3. CO_2 transport as bicarbonate

    - CO_2 in solution combines with water to form carbonic acid
    - Carbonic anhydrase
    - Zinc-containing enzyme within red blood cell
    - Carbonic acid ionizes into hydrogen ions and bicarbonate ions

$$CO_2 + H_2O \leftrightarrow H_2CO_3 \leftrightarrow H^+ + HCO_3^-$$

Question: Which of the three mechanisms transporting CO_2 transport the greatest amount of CO_2?

Chapter 11—Gas Exchange and Transport   161

Acid–Base Regulation:

Buffering:

- Acids (such as carbonic acid, H_2CO_3) dissociate in solution and release H^+ and HCO_3^-

$$CO_2 + H_2O \leftrightarrow H_2CO_3 \leftrightarrow H^+ + HCO_3^-$$

- Bases accept H^+ to form OH^- ions
- Buffers minimize changes in pH

Three mechanisms help regulate internal pH:

1. Chemical buffers consist of a weak acid and the salt of that acid.

   These act fast, but the *relative power of chemical buffers is small* compared to physiologic buffers!

2. Physiologic Buffers

   - Lungs regulate blood pH via CO_2 conversion to H_2CO_3 (fast acting effects)

$$CO_2 + H_2O \leftrightarrow H_2CO_3 \leftrightarrow H^+ + HCO_3^-$$

   Alveolar ventilation regulates $P{CO_2}$ which in turn affects blood pH via H_2CO_3

   - Increasing V_A lowers $PaCO_2$ which raises arterial pH (**respiratory alkalosis**).
   - Decreasing V_A raises $PaCO_2$ which lowers arterial pH (**respiratory acidosis**).

3. Kidneys

   - Kidneys regulate blood pH levels by secreting ammonia and H^+ into urine and reabsorbing chloride (Cl^-) and bicarbonate (HCO_3^-)
   - Active transport mechanisms (takes hours to days to have an effect

Gas Exchange and Hypoxemia:

Oxygenation is the process of transferring oxygen from the alveoli to the arterial blood.

Oxygenation requirements:

- Oxygen in alveoli
- Diffusion of oxygen to blood
- Perfusion of alveoli (blood flow)
- **Ventilation** (gas flow) and **perfusion** (blood flow) need to be matched.

Causes of hypoxemia (low arterial $P{O_2}$ or PaO_2):

- Hypoventilation
- Diffusion limitation

- Diffusion depends on pressure gradient!
- Alveolar–arterial P_{O_2} **(A–aP_{O_2}) difference** is a measure of the effectiveness of gas exchange
- Shunt
  - Refers to blood that never sees alveolar gas (i.e. no gas exchange)
  - In shunted blood the O_2 level remains the same as venous blood throughout the lung (e.g. capillary bed) and mixes into arterial blood.

    Examples include
    - Complete airway obstruction
    - Alveoli filled with debris (pneumonia, fluid)
    - Alveoli collapse
    - Blood flow through arterial or ventricular wall holes in the heart (i.e. right-to-left shunt)
    - Bronchial arteries and Thebesian veins (normal anatomy)
- Ventilation-perfusion (V/Q) mismatch
  - Gas and blood need to be in the same place at the same time!

Alveolar–arterial P_{O_2} difference (AaP_{O_2})

Hypoventilation	= normal $AaDO_2$
Diffusion limitation	= high $AaDO_2$
Shunt	= high $AaDO_2$
V/Q mismatch	= high $AaDO_2$

Exercise-induced arterial hypoxemia (EIAH) may occur in elite endurance athletes.

- Generally seen in male athletes with V_{O_2}max above 60 mL/kg/min.
- Because women have smaller airways, they may be more susceptible to EIAH at lower V_{O_2}max compared.
- Potential mechanisms include:
  - Relative hypoventilation
  - Failure to achieve equilibrium between alveoli and end-capillary P_{O_2} (i.e., diffusion limitation)
  - Shunting of blood flow bypassing alveolar capillaries (i.e. intrapulmonary shunts)
  - V/Q inequalities

Review Questions: Chapter 11

(For true and false questions that are false, indicate what would make the question true)

1. Define each of the following abbreviations:
   a. V̇E:
   b. V̇A:
   c. V̇O$_2$:
   d. V̇CO$_2$:
   e. PAO$_2$:
   f. PaO$_2$:
   g. PvO$_2$:
   h. SaO$_2$:
   i. FIO$_2$:

2. **True** or **False**: Henry's law states that gases diffuse from an area of high pressure to an area of low pressure.

3. What two factors that determine the diffusion of any gas?

4. State Dalton's Law:

5. a. In what two forms oxygen is transported in blood?

   b. Which of these two transports more O$_2$? Why?

6. **True** or **False**: Hemoglobin is approximately 75% saturated with O$_2$ at the level of the lung in a healthy individual who is at sea level.

Chapter 11—Gas Exchange and Transport   165

7. Fill in the values for P_{O_2} and CO_2 in the diagram below

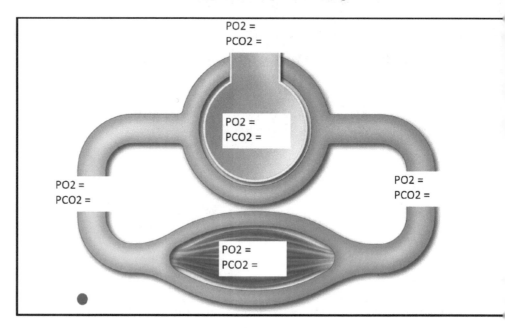

8. Myoglobin:
    a. Is an iron-containing globular protein in skeletal and cardiac muscle
    b. Stores O_2 intramuscularly
    c. Contains only 1 iron atom
    d. Releases O_2 at high P_{O_2}
        i. a, b, and c
        ii. b, c, and d
        iii. a, c, and d
        iv. a, b, and d
        v. All of these

9. List the *three* ways CO_2 is transported in the blood.
    1.
    2.
    3.

10. List the *three* mechanisms that help regulate pH of the body. Give an example of each.
    1.
    2.
    3.

11. Define hypoxemia:

12. A shunt could be caused by:
    a. Complete airway obstruction
    b. Pneumonia
    c. Alveolar collapse
    d. Blood flow through arterial or ventricular wall holes in the heart
       i. a, b, and c
       ii. b, c, and d
       iii. a, c, and d
       iv. a, b, and d
       v. all of these

13. **True** or **False**: EIAH occurs most frequently in people whose V_{O_2} max is less than 60 mL/kg/min.

14. **True** or **False**: The resting arterial minus mixed venous oxygen difference (a–V_{O_2} difference) of 4 to 5 mL of oxygen indicates that approximately 50% of the available O_2 has been released from hemoglobin.

15. What is 2-3 diphophoglycerate (2,3-DPG)?
    a. How is it produced?
    b. How does it affect the oxyhemoglobin curve?

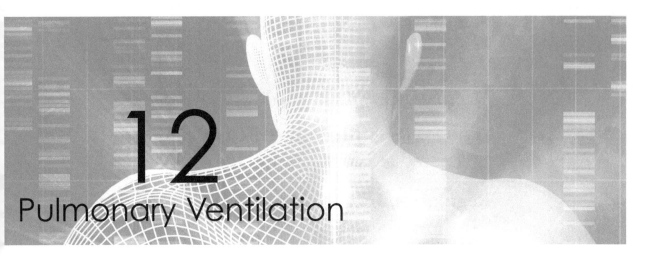

12
Pulmonary Ventilation

CONTROL OF VENTILATION

Brain is the central controller.

- Cortex exerts voluntary control on respiration
- Hypothalamus and limbic system exert emotional/stress control on respiration
- Brainstem exerts autonomic (or involuntary) control on respiration

Autonomic control is the primary control of respiration and requires several levels of sensory input

- Chemoreceptors (chemical control)
  - P_{O_2}
  - P_{CO_2}
  - $[H^+]$
- Lung receptors
  - Irritant
  - Stretch
- Other receptors
  - Baroreceptors in arterial system (senses blood pressure)
  - Temperature
  - Pain
  - Muscle receptors

Central chemoreceptors are on the brain stem (known as the **medullary respiratory centers**)

- Responds to CSF pH (effected by P_{CO_2})

Peripheral chemoreceptors are located in aorta arch and carotid arteries

- Monitor P_{CO_2} and P_{O_2} and pH
- Respond to hypoxia!
- Transmits via glossopharyngeal nerve (cranial nerve IX)

Hyperventilation and Breath Holding

- Hyperventilation decreases alveolar and arterial P_{CO_2} to very low levels.

Regulation of Ventilation during Exercise

- Chemical control does not entirely account for increased ventilation during exercise
- Nonchemical control seems to play a major role:
  - Neurogenic factors (cortical influence and peripheral influence)
  - Temperature has little influence on respiratory rate during exercise

Integrated Regulation of Ventilation during Exercise

Phase I (beginning of exercise)

- Neurogenic stimuli from cortex increase respiration

Phase II (After about 20 seconds, V_E rises exponentially to reach steady state).

- Central command
- Peripheral chemoreceptors

Phase III (during steady state exercise)

- Fine tuning of steady-state ventilation through peripheral sensory feedback mechanisms.

Recovery

- An abrupt decline in ventilation reflects removal of central command and input from receptors in active muscle
- Slower recovery phase from gradual metabolic, chemical, and thermal adjustments

Ventilation in Steady State Exercise

During **light** to **moderate** exercise:

- Ventilation increases *linearly* with O_2 consumption and CO_2 production
- This relationship is termed **"Ventilatory Equivalent"** (V_E/VO_2)
- Normal $V_E/VO_2 = 20$ to 25 in adults (up to 32 in children)

Ventilation in Non-Steady State Exercise

Above moderate exercise:

- V_E rises sharply and disproportionately with O_2 consumption during exercise. This is termed "**Ventilatory Threshold**"

- V_E/VO_2 = increases during exercise (up to 35 to 40)
- Sodium bicarbonate in the blood buffers almost all of the lactate generated via glycolysis

$$La + NaHCO_3 \leftrightarrow NaLa + H_2CO_3$$

- As lactate is buffered, CO_2 is regenerated from the bicarbonate, stimulating ventilation.

$$H_2CO_3 \leftrightarrow CO_2 + H_2O$$

- **Lactate threshold**
  - Describes highest V_{O2} exercise intensity with less than a 1 mM/L increase in blood lactate above resting level.
- **Onset of Blood Lactate Accumulation (OBLA)**
  - OBLA differs with exercise mode due to muscle mass being activated.
  - OBLA occurs at lower exercise levels during cycling of arm-crank exercise.

Specificity of OBLA

- Useful to predict exercise performance (i.e., maximum intensity a person can maintain for a prolonged period).
- OBLA differs with exercise mode due to muscle mass being activated.
  - OBLA occurs at lower exercise levels during cycling of arm-crank exercise.

  However, there is some independence between OBLA and VO_2

- Factors influencing ability to sustain a percentage of aerobic capacity without lactate accumulation.
  - Muscle fiber type
  - Capillary density
  - Mitochondria size and number
  - Muscle enzyme concentration

Effects of intense exercise

- During exercise, pH decreases as VCO_2 and lactate production increase.
- Low levels of pH are not well tolerated and need to be quickly buffered.

Energy cost of breathing

- At rest and during light exercise, the O_2 cost of breathing is small.
- During maximal exercise, the respiratory muscles require a significant portion of total blood flow (up to 15%).

Respiratory disease

- Chronic obstructive pulmonary disease (COPD) may triple the O_2 cost of breathing at rest.
- This severely limits exercise capacity in COPD patients.

Chapter 12—Pulmonary Ventilation   171

Does ventilation limit aerobic power and endurance?

- Healthy individuals overbreathe at higher levels of O_2 consumption.

- At max exercise, there usually is a breathing reserve.

- Ventilation in healthy individuals is generally not the limiting factor in exercise.

Cigarette smoking

- Increased airway resistance

- Increased rates of asthma and related symptoms

- Smoking increases reliance on CHO during exercise

- Smoking blunts HR response to exercise

Ventilation in Hypoxia

- Exposure to hypoxia results in **respiratory alkalosis** due to **hypoxic ventilatory drive (HVR)**

$$\downarrow P_b \quad \Leftrightarrow \quad \downarrow PaO_2 \quad \Leftrightarrow \quad \uparrow V_E \quad \Leftrightarrow \quad \downarrow PaCO_2 \quad \Leftrightarrow \quad \uparrow pH$$

*Remember this hyperventilation is being driven by **peripheral chemoreceptors!***

Symptoms of respiratory alkalosis (overlap with acute mountain sickness)

- Tackcardia

- Numbness and tingling in extremities

- Lethargy and confusion

- Light headedness

- Nausea

- Anxiety, fear

- Seizures

- In the brain, **central chemoreceptors** sense,

$\downarrow PaCO_2 \quad \Leftrightarrow \quad \uparrow CSF$ pH, which in turn tries to $\downarrow V_E$

(this actually acts to "brake" or reduce the HVR response to ventilation)

- After 1 to 3 days in hypoxia (this process is called **acclimatization**)

  - Choroid plexus excretes $HCO_3^- \quad \Leftrightarrow \quad$ CSF pH$\downarrow$ (to normal)

  - Central CO_2 sensitivity is reset to lower level

  - "Releases" the brake on ventilation, so now HVR is able to further increase V_E

Review Questions: Chapter 12

(For true and false questions that are false, indicate what would make the question true)

1. The normal respiratory cycle is governed by the medial portion of the
    _____.

2. Inspiratory neurons activate the _____ and _____ to cause
    the lungs to inflate.

3. What two factors cause the inspiratory neurons to cease firing?

    a.

    b.

4. Under resting conditions, how is exhalation normally initiated? Is this
    different during exercise, if so, how?

5. How is the hypothalamus involved in the respiratory cycle?

6. At rest, _____ is the greatest respiratory stimulator. Small increas-
    es in _____ result in large increases in minute ventilation.

7. Peripheral chemoreceptors monitor and respond to what?

8. **True** or **False**: Hyperventilation can decrease alveolar and arterial
    P_{O_2} which allows an individual to hold his or her breath longer.

9. What are the three phases of ventilation response to moderate exer-
    cise? What happens in each phase?

    a.

    b.

    c.

10. What happens to ventilation during recovery?

11. How is the ventilatory equivalent calculated?

12. **True** or **False**: The ventilatory equivalent increases linearly from rest
    to max exercise.

13. Define the ventilatory threshold?

Chapter 12—Pulmonary Ventilation   173

14.   What causes the ventilatory threshold during exercise?

15.   The OBLA:

    a. Is the point where the body first begins to produce lactate.

    b. Differs with exercise mode due to muscle mass being activated.

    c. Can be trained to occur at a higher relative percentage of one's maximal aerobic capacity.

    d. Occurs at lower exercise levels during cycling of arm-crank exercise.

       i. a, b, and c

      ii. b, c, and d

     iii. a, c, and d

     iv. a, b, and d

      v. all of these

16.   How does acidosis affect respiration?

    a. How does it relate to CO_2 and carbonic acid formation?

    b. How does it relate to lactate formation?

    c. How does it relate to ketone formation?

17.   You should know how the occurrence of COPD affects:

    a. Expiratory resistance?

    b. Energy cost of breathing?

    c. How does this relate to the ability to perform exercise?

18.   What is EIAH?

When does it typically occur?

Chapters 10, 11 & 12

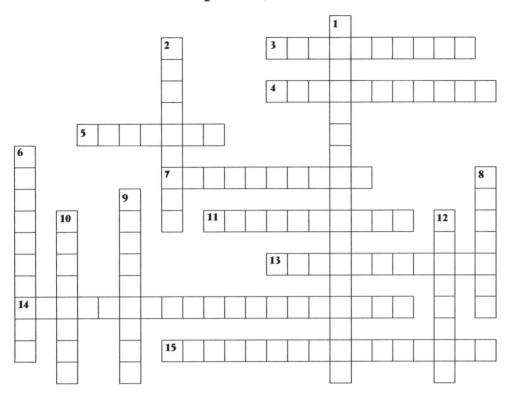

ACROSS

3 The iron-protein pigment in the red blood cell.
4 Volume of air inspired or expired per breath.
5 Area of the brain that governs the normal respiratory cycle.
7 Lipoprotein mixture that reduces alveolar surface tension.
11 Percentage of centrifuged whole blood for red blood cells and plasma.
13 The process during which the diaphragm muscle contracts and flattens.
14 Maximum volume inspired following tidal expiration.
15 Conscious increases in ventilation above normal breathing.

DOWN

1 Volume in lungs after maximum inspiration.
2 Referese to increase pH.
6 The process that is passive during rest.
8 Shortness of breath.
9 Large dome-shaped sheet of striated musculo-fibrous tissue.
10 Governs gas diffusion through the alveolar membrane.
12 Refers to increased H+ concentration.

Chapter 12—Pulmonary Ventilation   175

SECTION ONE: LABORATORY ASSIGNMENTS
Unit One Laboratories

Name: _____

Three-Day Food Diary and Nutritional Assessment

Objective of this lab: To record everything that you eat and drink for three consecutive days in order to perform a nutritional analysis.

Key Concepts:

1. Understand how to accurately measure and /or quantify the types and amounts of food and drink that you consume over the course of a three-day period.

2. Understand how to accurately record and enter dietary consumption information into a nutritional database and analyze the nutritional breakdown of your diet.

3. Understand how to compare your average nutritional intake to the U.S. Department of Agriculture recommendations.

Instructions

Record everything that you eat and drink on the following forms for three consecutive days (Thursday, Friday, and Saturday, ideally). This includes all meals, snacks, nibbling, sampling, sodas, cocktails, and so on. Always record in your food logs immediately after having a meal, snack, or drink. Here are some helpful hints for entering foods to make sure your nutritional analysis is more accurate.

1. **Only record one food item per line.**

   Example: Regular coffee 1 c.
           Creamer 1 Tb.
           Sugar 1 tsp.

2. **Indicate amounts**

   - Use measuring spoons for jelly, sugar, syrup, gravy, salad dressing, mayonnaise, butter, and margarine. 3 teaspoon (tsp.) = 1 tablespoon (Tb.)

   - Use measuring cups for vegetables, rice, noodles, cereals, soups, stews, casseroles, ice cream, Jell-O, and canned fruits. A bowl of soup or a plate of spaghetti should be entered in cups. 1 cup (c.) = 8 ounces.

   - Use ounces or dimensions for meat, fish, poultry, cheese, pizza, cakes, pies, cookies, etc. Specify a piece of pie/cake as 1/8, 1/6, etc. portion.

   - Use number and size (small, medium, large) for breads, rolls, raw fruits, hot dogs, lunchmeat, crackers, chips, and candy.

Unit One Laboratories   177

- If you are entering foods by their weight, enter only the weight for the edible portion; do not include the bone, skin, etc.

3. **Indicate how the food was prepared.**

   - Specify if the food is fresh, cooked, or prepared from can/box. If canned, specify if it was canned in juice, water, or light or heavy syrup. Did you use the solids and liquid, or drain it first? Example: Baked or fried, trimmed or untrimmed, poultry skin removed or left on.

   - Specify if it was cooked from fresh, frozen, or canned. Was it boiled, baked, fried, steamed, broiled, or roasted? If it was prepared from a mix, did you add water or milk? If you added milk, did you add skim, 1%, 2%, or whole milk?

4. **Indicate fats used in cooking and how much on another line.** Example: Fried 1 tsp. corn oil

5. **Indicate whether the food was eaten at home or in a restaurant.**

   - Ask your wait staff the portion sizes. If you record a menu weight, be sure to indicate the menu or raw weight on your record. If you do not know the weight of a food, use dimensions to describe the food. You cannot use dimensions for foods that are not solids (e.g., green beans, salads, peas). Use cups to describe these foods. You can use dimensions for solid foods (e.g., steak, baked potato, submarine roll, luncheon meats, or cheeses).

6. **Include the labels of the food eaten** (especially if the product is not from one of the well-known manufacturers).

7. **Recipes and condiments:** For combination dish, identify the major ingredients or components. For a sandwich, enter the components. Be sure to specify the type of bread—white, whole wheat, or wheat (part whole wheat), cracked wheat, etc. Example: 1 c. cooked pasta, 1/2 c. tomato sauce, 2 Tb. Parmesan, etc.

Food Diary

Day of week and date: <u>Thursday, April 19</u>

	Time	Amount (Specify cup, tsp., Tb., etc.)	List food or drink with details
1	6:30 am	1 cup	Regular coffee, black, no cream or sugar
2		1/2	English muffin, 100% whole wheat, toasted
3		2 Tb.	Unsweetened applesauce
4	10:00 am	1 large	Apple
5	12 noon	2 slices	White bread
6		2 oz.	Oscar Mayer bologna
7		2 Tb.	Mayonnaise
8		1/2 cup	Deli potato salad
9	3:15 pm	2 medium	Choc. chip cookie
10		1 cup	2% milk
11	6:30 pm	1 medium	Chicken breast
12		2 Tb.	Parmesan cheese
13		1/2 cup	Tomato sauce
14		2 cup	Garden salad
15		1/4 cup	Light blue cheese dressing
16		1/2 cup	Buttered steamed broccoli
17		1 medium	Dinner roll
18		1 1/2 tsp.	Parkay margarine
19		1/8 portion	Choc. ice cream cake
20		2 Tb.	Cherry topping
21		2 cups	Decaff. coffee
22		12 oz.	Diet Sprite
23			
24			
25			
26			
27			
28			

Day of Week and Date: _____

	Time	Amount (Specify cup, tsp., Tb., etc.)	List food or drink with details
1			
2			
3			
4			
5			
6			
7			
8			
9			
10			
11			
12			
13			
14			
15			
16			
17			
18			
19			
20			
21			
22			
23			
24			
25			
26			
27			
28			
29			
30			

Day of Week and Date: _____

	Time	Amount (Specify cup, tsp., Tb., etc.)	List food or drink with details
1			
2			
3			
4			
5			
6			
7			
8			
9			
10			
11			
12			
13			
14			
15			
16			
17			
18			
19			
20			
21			
22			
23			
24			
25			
26			
27			
28			
29			
30			

Day of Week and Date: _____

	Time	Amount (Specify cup, tsp., Tb., etc.)	List food or drink with details
1			
2			
3			
4			
5			
6			
7			
8			
9			
10			
11			
12			
13			
14			
15			
16			
17			
18			
19			
20			
21			
22			
23			
24			
25			
26			
27			
28			
29			
30			

Questions

1. What is your average daily caloric intake? Compare this to the recommended daily caloric intake.

2. What percentage of your calories are from carbohydrate? Protein? Fat? Compare your results to the USDA recommendations.

3. What percent of calories should come from saturated fatty acids? What percent of your diet is made up of saturated fatty acids? Discuss the significance of saturated fatty acids in the diet.

4. What is your average daily sodium intake? Is your sodium intake above or below recommended levels? Discuss the significance of too much or too little sodium in the diet.

5. What percentage of your caloric intake is from sugars? How does your intake of simple sugars compare to the USDA recommendations? What are the concerns with consuming too much simple sugar?

Unit One Laboratories   183

6. Discuss what it means to consume nutrient-dense foods. Based on your diet analysis, do you feel that you consume sufficient nutrient-dense foods? How might you modify your diet in order to consume more nutrient-dense foods?

Wingate Cycle Ergometer Test

Objective of this lab: To perform a supramaximal Wingate cycle ergometer test to measure peak anaerobic power, mean anaerobic power, total work, fatigue index, and peak blood lactate concentrations.

Key Concepts:

1. Ability to accurately determine and apply workloads needed to perform the Wingate test based upon the test subject's gender and body weight.

2. Ability to proficiently administer the supramaximal Wingate test so that measures of peak anaerobic power, total work, and fatigue index can be obtained.

3. Understand the contribution of various energy metabolism pathways that are involved during the Wingate test.

4. Understand the rational and usefulness of the Wingate test.

Instructions

1. Measure and record the subjects body weight: _____lbs/2.2 = _____ kg

2. Calculate the force (resistance) needed to perform the Wingate test using the following equation:

   Body weight (kg) * 0.075 = resistance needed for the weight tray

   _____* 0.075 = _____kg

3. Test subject should adjust seat height so that the knee has a slight bend (5-15 degrees when ball of foot is on the pedal).

4. The subject MUST remain SEATED during the duration of the test!!!

Wingate Test Protocol		
Period	**Time**	**Activity**
Warm up	5 minutes	Cycle at low to moderate intensity interspersed with four or five all-out sprints of 4-6 seconds with prescribed force.
Recovery	5 minutes	Rest or cycle slowly against zero resistance.
Acceleration	5-15 seconds	With no resistance, have subject reach maximal rpm.
Wingate	30 seconds	Cycle at highest possible rpm at target resistance. Perform a second blood lactate measurement.
Cool down	2-5 minutes	Cycle at low to moderate intensity (50 rpm with 1 kg resistance).

Source: Table adapted from Bar-Or, O. (1978). A new anaerobic capacity test: Characteristics applications. Proceedings of the 21st World Congress in Sports Medicine at Brasilia.

Questions

1. Discuss what energy-producing pathways are likely the predominant pathways throughout the 30 seconds of the actual Wingate test. For example, during the first several seconds of the actual Wingate test, the ATP that is being utilized is likely coming from where? As the Wingate test progresses (10–30 seconds of actual Wingate test), what energy pathways are the predominant sources of energy?

2. a. Peak anaerobic power is based on the highest power level averaged over a specified time period (usually 2–5 seconds). At what time during the actual Wingate test would you expect to see peak anaerobic power occur?

   b. Record and identify when the absolute peak anaerobic power occurred during your test. The units of measure should be watts (W).

3. a. To interpret the results, the absolute peak anaerobic power is often divided by the subject's body weight in kg. This is referred to as the *relative peak anaerobic power output*. Calculate your relative peak anaerobic power output.

   b. Discuss the advantages of calculating the relative peak anaerobic power output.

4. Some research suggests that a resistance of 7.5% of the subject's body weight may not be the optimal force needed to measure peak power output. Explain how increasing or decreasing the resistance may yield higher power output. What factors contribute to peak power output, and how will these factors be affected by increasing or decreasing the resistance?

Unit One Laboratories   187

5. The fatigue index represents the degree of fatigue throughout the course of the actual Wingate test. A higher fatigue index represents a decreased ability to maintain the power level over the course of the test due to neuromuscular fatigue. The fatigue index is calculated as the percent decrease in power (p) from the highest power to the lowest power.

Fatigue index (%) = [(Highest power – Lowest power)/Highest power] * 100

Calculate your fatigue index from your test data.

6. Discuss some sporting events in which having above-average peak power output and a lower fatigue index may increase sport performance.

7. A popular nutritional supplement utilized by individuals hoping to improve peak power output is creatine monohydrate. Using what you know about metabolism, what is the rationale for using this supplement?

8 Discuss how the blood lactate is being produced and why there is lactate in the blood even at rest.

9. If three 20 year old male subjects – (1) is sedentary, (2) is an endurance-trained athlete, and (3) is a resistance-trained power lifter-completed the same Wingate test, which would you expect to obtain the highest blood lactate levels and why? Discuss the differences you would expect to see in absolute peak power and relative peak power for the three individuals..

Unit Two Laboratories

Name: _____

Estimation of Cardiorespiratory Fitness from Field and Submaximal Exercise Test Laboratory

Objective of this lab: To perform commonly utilized validated laboratory and field exercise tests for the purpose of determining cardiorespiratory fitness capacity.

Key Concepts:

1. Ability to safely and correctly administer the following exercise tests: YMCA Submaximal Cycle Test, Submaximal Bruce Treadmill Test, Rockport 1-Mile Walk Test, Cooper 1.5-Mile Run Test, George Jog Test, and Cooper 12-Minute Walk/Run Test.

2. Demonstrate how measures of cardiorespiratory fitness (Max VO_2) can be predicted from the highest work rate achieved during a submaximal exercise test.

3. Understand potential sources of error in submaximal exercise tests when predicting Max VO_2.

4. Understand the advantages and disadvantages of performing submaximal exercise tests for the purpose of predicting cardiorespiratory fitness.

5. Understand the advantages and disadvantages of performing field tests versus laboratory-based tests of cardiorespiratory fitness.

Cardiorespiratory Fitness from the Field

Rockport 1-Mile Walk Test

1. **Walk** as fast as possible for 1 mile (preferably on a flat surface).

2. Record finishing time.

3. Obtain HR in the last minute.

4. Calculate VO_2 from the specific equation:

$$VO_{2max} \text{ (mL} \cdot \text{kg}^{-1} \cdot \text{min}^{-1}) = 132.853 - 0.1692 \text{ (body mass in kg)}$$
$$- 0.3877 \text{ (age in years)} + 6.315 \text{ (gender)} - 3.2649 \text{ (time in minutes)}$$
$$- 0.1565 \text{ (HR)}$$

  *gender = 0 for female and 1 for male
  *HR = HR taken at the end of the walk.

Cooper 1.5-Mile Run Test

1. Run 1.5 miles in the shortest time possible.

2. Record finishing time.

Unit Two Laboratories 189

3. Calculate VO_2 from the specific equation:

$$VO_{2max} \; (mL \cdot kg^{-1} \cdot min^{-1}) = 3.5 + 483/(\text{time in minutes})$$

George Jog Test

1. Jog 1 mile at a comfortable pace.

   a. The time for the mile should be greater than 8 minutes for males and greater than 9 minutes for females

2. Record finishing time.

3. Obtain HR at the end of jog.

4. Calculate VO_2 from the specific equation:

$$VO_{2max} \; (mL \cdot kg^{-1} \cdot min^{-1}) = 100.5 + (8.344 \times \text{gender})$$
$$- (0.0744 \times \text{weight}) - (1.438 \times \text{mile time}) - (0.1928 \times \text{heart rate})$$

*gender = 1 for male; 0 for female
*weight = pounds
*time = minutes and fraction of minutes (14:30 = 14.5 minutes)

Cooper 12 minute Walk/Run Test

1. Cover the greatest amount of distance in the 12 minute time period

2. Record final distance.

3. Calculate VO_2 from the specific equation:

$$VO_{2max} \; (mL \cdot kg^{-1} \cdot min^{-1}) = (35.97 \times \text{miles}) - 11.29$$

Submax Questions

1. List and explain three sources if error that may contribute to errors in estimating VO2 max from these submax tests.

2. List and describe three benefits to field-testing compared to laboratory testing.

3. What is the difference between absolute VO2 and relative VO2?

YMCA Submaximal Cycle Test

1. Have test subject complete a physical activity readiness questionnaire (PAR-Q) and review the responses with your laboratory instructor.

2. Place a Polar heart-rate monitor band around the chest and the HR monitor on the wrist. Verify the HR monitor is displaying accurate HR readings by palpating the radial artery and counting the HR.

3. Position the seat of the Monarch cycle ergometer to allow for a 5- to 15-degree bend of the knee of the subject.

4. Review the following protocol with the test subject and verify correct workloads can be set on the Monarch cycle ergometer by having the subject pedal at a speed of **50 rpm. Recall:** Work = Force * Distance

   a. 1st stage 150 kg·m·min^{-1} = Force (kg) * (50 rpm * 6 m·rev^{-1})

$$Force (kg) = \frac{150 \text{ kg·m·in}^{-1}}{300 \text{ m·min}^{-1}}$$

   Force (kg) = 0.5 kg

1st stage = 150 kg·m·min^{-1}				
	HR < 80	HR: 80–89	HR: 90–100	HR > 100
2nd Stage	750 kg·m·min^{-1} (2.5 kg)	600 kg·m·min^{-1} (2.0 kg)	450 kg·m·min^{-1} (1.5 kg)	300 kg·m·min^{-1} (1.0 kg)
3rd Stage	900 kg·m·min^{-1} (3.0 kg)	750 kg·m·min^{-1} (2.5 kg)	600 kg·m·min^{-1} (2.0 kg)	450 kg·m·min^{-1} (1.5 kg)
4th Stage	1050 kg·m·min^{-1} (3.5 kg)	900 kg·m·min^{-1} (3.0 kg)	700 kg·m·min^{-1} (2.5 kg)	600 kg·m·min^{-1} (2.0 kg)

5. Each stage should last 3 minutes with heart rates being recorded at the end of each minute. Ensure that steady state HR is achieved (≤ 6 bpm) between the last 2 minutes of each stage.

6. Record rating of perceived exertion at the end of each stage.

7. The test should be terminated when the subject reaches 85% of age-predicted maximal heart rate, fails to conform to the exercise protocol, develops adverse signs, and /or symptoms, requests to stop, or experiences any emergency situation.

8. Allow subject to cool down by continuing to pedal against a workload of 150 kg·m·min^{-1}.

YMCA SUBMAXIMAL CYCLE TEST DATA SHEET

Subject's name: _____   **Age:** _____   **Weight:** _____

Resting heart rate: _____

85% Age-predicted MAXHR = (220 − Age) = _____ *** 0.85 =** _____

STAGE	Heart Rate	RPE
150 kg·m·min^{-1}	_____ _____ _____	_____ _____ _____
kg·m·min^{-1}	_____ _____ _____	_____ _____ _____
kg·m·min^{-1}	_____ _____ _____	_____ _____ _____
kg·m·min^{-1}	_____ _____ _____	_____ _____ _____

Questions

1. Predict the Max VO_2 using the supplied HR – Workload graph. Convert the predicted absolute maximal VO_2 obtained to the predicted relative maximal VO_2. Remember, relative VO_2 has units of $ml\cdot kg^{-1}\cdot min^{-1}$.

2. Calculate the predicted Max VO_2 using the calculation of the slope of the HR – Workload relationship, where slope $(m) = (VO_22 - VO_21)/(HR2 - HR1)$ and predicted Max $VO_2 = m(HR_{max} - HR2) + VO_22$. Recall that the VO_2 for any given work rate on a cycle ergometer can be calculated by the equation:

    $VO_2 = [(1.8 * $ work rate$)/$Body weight$] + 7$

3. Classify this cycle ergometer test (lab vs. field test, submaximal vs. maximal test) and discuss the advantages and disadvantages of these types of tests.

4. Discuss the sources of error in predicting Max VO_2 from this type of test.

Unit Two Laboratories   197

Graded Maximal Exercise Testing and Determination of Ventilatory Threshold and Ventilatory Equivalents

Objective of this lab: To perform a symptom-limited maximal graded exercise test with breath-by-breath open-circuit spirometry for the determination of VO_{2Max} and ventilatory threshold.

Key Concepts:

1. Ability to utilize breath-by-breath open-circuit spirometry during a symptom-limited maximal graded exercise test.

2. Understand the procedures necessary for successful calibration and test operation of the metabolic system.

3. Interpret and explain breath-by-breath changes at rest and during exercise for FeO_2, $FeCO_2$, VO_2, VCO_2, RER, Ve, Vt, Ve/VO_2, and Ve/VCO_2.

4. Ability to identify the ventilatory threshold using the intercept of S1 and S2 of the V-slope graph.

5. Ability to verify the ventilatory threshold using the ventilatory equivalents, Ve/VO_2 and Ve/VCO_2.

6. Ability to identify the suspected period of isocapnic buffering and respiratory compensation using the ventilatory equivalents.

Instructions

1. Have test subject complete a physical activity readiness questionnaire (PAR-Q) and review the responses with your laboratory instructor.

2. Place a Polar heart rate monitor band around the chest and the HR monitor on the wrist. Verify the HR monitor is displaying accurate HR readings by palpating the radial artery and counting the HR.

3. Calibrate the breath-by-breath metabolic system according to manufacturer instructions.

4. Fit face mask and head gear of the metabolic system onto the subject.

5. Enter test subject's data into the metabolic system and choose maximal treadmill test as the type of test.

6. Select and perform the Bruce protocol.

7. Record rating of perceived exertion at the end of each stage.

8. Encourage participant to continue to push him- or herself to volitional fatigue.

9. The test should be terminated when the subject requests to stop, fails to conform to the exercise protocol, develops adverse signs and/or symptoms, or experiences any emergency situation.

Unit Two Laboratories   199

10. When the test is terminated, immediately begin the active recovery by clicking on the cool-down button and allow the subject to continue walking at 0% elevation and 1.5 mph.

11. Remove subject's face mask during the active recovery.

12. Upon completion of test, print off the ventilatory threshold graph, the summary report, the 9-panel report, and the text report from the reports tab.

Questions

1. What are VO_2 and VO_2 Max?

2. How can VO_2 max be improved?

3. Explain 4 different factors that affect VO_2 max.

4. Name the 4 criteria that lets us know if someone is at max (GIVE EXAMPLES OF EACH).

Unit Three Laboratories

Name: _____

Anthropometry Laboratory

Objective of this lab: The purpose of this lab is to provide hands-on knowledge of certain anatomical surface landmarks and basic biomechanical anthropometric measurement techniques.

Key Concepts:

1. Students will palpate common lower extremity landmarks.

2. Students will perform two common leg-length measurement techniques and discuss differences between them.

3. Students will display an ability to assess quadriceps angle.

4. Students will use a search engine such as PubMed to find a peer-reviewed scientific research article dealing with anthropometry. Students will also interpret the results of this research article.

5. Students will assess passive and active knee range of motion and understand the differences between the two measurement techniques.

Equipment:

Goniometer

Anthropometric tape

String

Non-toxic marker to mark body landmarks

Attire:

Students will arrive at the laboratory session in a short sleeve T-shirt and shorts. No shoes are to be worn during the laboratory; however, low-cut socks (i.e. beneath the ankle) are permitted.

Procedures:

Students will organize themselves into groups of 3 students each. Each person will perform measurements on another student in the group, while the third student will record these measurements. After the measurements are performed, students will rotate roles so that each student has an opportunity to be the measurer, subject, and data recorder in each station before moving to the next station.

Measurements

1. <u>True Leg Length</u>

   a. Instruct the subject to lay supine (i.e., face up) on the floor of the laboratory.

   b. Instruct the subject to flex the knees, sliding the feet along the floor to bring the feet closer to the body.

Unit Three Laboratories   203

c. To get the pelvis in a neutral position, instruct the subject to lift the bottom off of the floor by extending the hips and pushing up. The subject can then lower him-or herself back to the floor. From here on, the subject is in a relaxed position and the measurer is going to do all of the work.

d. Grab the subject's ankles and pull them down until the subject is lying in a natural supine position again.

e. Find the center of each of the medial malleoli. Make a small dot with the non-toxic marker in the center of each of the medial malleoli.

f. Palpate the subject's left anterior superior iliac spine (ASIS). Put the "0" of the anthropometric measuring tape on the left ASIS and stretch it to the mark on the left medial malleolus. Record the true leg length for the left side on the data sheet.

g. Repeat two more times to ensure the accuracy of your measurement.

h. Repeat steps d–g on the right side and record the true leg length for the right side on the data sheet.

2. Functional Leg Length

a. Instruct the subject to lay supine (i.e., face up) on the floor of the laboratory.

b. Instruct the subject to flex the knees, sliding the feet along the floor to bring the feet closer to the body.

c. To get the pelvis in a neutral position, instruct the subject to lift the bottom off of the floor by extending the hips and pushing up. The subject can then lower him- or herself back to the floor. From here on, the subject is in a relaxed position and the measurer is going to do all of the work.

d. Grab the subject's ankles and pull them down until the subject is lying in a natural supine position again.

e. Locate the subject's umbilicus. Put the "0" of the anthropometric measuring tape on the umbilicus and stretch it to the mark on the left medial malleolus. Record the functional leg length for the left side on the data sheet.

f. Repeat two more times to ensure the accuracy of your measurement.

g. Repeat steps e–f on the right side and record the functional leg length for the right side on the data sheet.

3. Qualitative Assessment of a Leg-Length Discrepancy

a. Place your thumbs over the subject's left and right medial malleoli.

b. Look at the difference in your thumb position between the left and right malleoli.

c. Notice if you would consider the person to have a difference in leg length. Write down your results here for future use in this lab.

Notes:

4. Quadriceps Angle (Q-Angle)

   a. Instruct the subject to lay supine (i.e., face up) on the floor of the laboratory.

   b. Instruct the subject to flex the knees, sliding the feet along the floor to bring the feet closer to the body.

   c. To get the pelvis in a neutral position, instruct the subject to lift the bottom off of the floor by extending the hips and pushing up. The subject can then lower him- or herself back to the floor. From here on, the subject is in a relaxed position and the measurer is going to do all of the work.

   d. Grab the subject's ankles and pull them down until the subject is lying in a natural supine position again.

   e. Using a non-toxic marker, place a dot in the center of the subject's left patella.

   f. Using a non-toxic marker, place a dot on the subject's left tibial tuberosity.

   g. Palpate the subject's left ASIS. Get a piece of string, and ask the subject to hold the end of the string on the left ASIS.

   h. Stretch this string until it passes directly above the mark placed at the center of the patella. Give the other end of this string to the recorder and ask him or her to hold it there.

   i. Using the subject and recorder as helpers, stretch a second piece of string above the marks made on the tibial tuberosity and the patella. Give the proximal end to the subject to hold, and give the distal end to the recorder. Make sure that they are holding the string so that the string still passes above the tibial tuberosity and the center of the patella.

   j. Using the goniometer, record the angle between the two strings.

   k. Repeat two more times to ensure the accuracy of your measurement.

   l. Repeat steps e–k on the right side and record the quadriceps angle for the right side on the data sheet.

5. Active Knee Range of Motion

   a. Instruct the subject to lay supine (i.e., face up) on the floor of the laboratory.

   b. Make sure that the left hip is in zero degrees of abduction/adduction and rotation.

   c. Using the non-toxic marker, place a dot on the left-side greater trochanter.

   d. Place another dot on the center of the left lateral epicondyle of the femur.

   e. Place a third dot on the left lateral malleolus.

Unit Three Laboratories   205

f. Align the goniometer so that the center hole in the goniometer is aligned with the knee joint mark, the proximal arm is pointing toward the mark on the greater trochanter, and the distal arm is pointing toward the mark on the lateral malleolus.

g. Ask the subject to extend the knee as much as possible. Hold the goniometer securely to the subject's leg so that it does not move out of position.

h. Record the active knee extension (°) result in your data table.

i. Ask the subject to pull the foot in toward the buttocks while keeping the foot flat on the floor. Hold the goniometer securely to the subject's leg so that it does not move out of position.

j. When the subject cannot pull the foot in any closer, record the active knee flexion (°) result in your data table.

k. Repeat steps f–j two more times to ensure accuracy of your measurement.

l. Repeat steps b–k on the right side and record the active knee extension and flexion results for the right side on the data sheet.

6. Passive Knee Range of Motion

a. Instruct the subject to lay supine (i.e., face up) on the floor of the laboratory.

b. Make sure that the left hip is in zero degrees of abduction/adduction and rotation.

c. Align the goniometer so that the center hole in the goniometer is aligned with the knee joint mark, the proximal arm is pointing toward the mark on the greater trochanter, and the distal arm is pointing toward the mark on the lateral malleolus.

d. Hold the goniometer securely to the subject's leg so that it does not move out of position. Ask the subject to extend the knee as much as possible. Then gently apply a little bit more force until you reach the end point of the range of motion.

e. Record the passive knee extension (°) result in your data table.

f. Hold the goniometer securely to the subject's leg so that it does not move out of position. Ask the subject to pull the foot in toward the buttocks while keeping the foot flat on the floor. When the end point in the range of motion is reached, gently apply more force until you reach the true end point of the range of motion.

g. Record the passive knee extension (°) result in your data table.

h. Repeat steps c–g two more times to ensure the accuracy of your measurement.

i. Repeat steps b–h on the right side and record the passive knee extension and flexion results for the right side on the data sheet.

206   Unit Three Laboratories

ANTHROPOMETRY LABORATORY DATA SHEET

Group Members: _____ (Measurer)

_____ (Subject)

_____ (Recorder)

Measurement	Left		Right		L-R Difference
	Individual Trials	**Average**	**Individual Trials**	**Average**	
True Leg Length (cm)					
Functional Leg Length (cm)					
Quadriceps Angle (°)					
					Knee ROM
Active Knee Extension (°)					Left ROM:
Active Knee Flexion (°)					Right ROM:
Passive Knee Extension (°)					Left ROM:
Passive Knee Flexion (°)					Right ROM:

Unit Three Laboratories   207

Questions

1. In the last column of the measurement sheet, calculate the difference between the left and right legs for the true leg-length assessment. Is there a leg length discrepancy (i.e., > 2.0 cm) in terms of true leg length?

2. In the last column of the measurement sheet, calculate the difference between the left and right legs for the functional leg-length assessment. Is there a leg length discrepancy (i.e., > 2.0 cm) in terms of functional leg length?

3. The true leg-length measurement and the functional leg-length measurements use different anatomical landmarks. Considering this, what biomechanical/anatomical factors may be related to differences in these measurements?

4. How well does your qualitative assessment of the subject's leg length agree with the results from questions 1 and 2?

5. A normal quadriceps angle is: 14 ± 3 degrees for males and 17 ± 3 degrees for women. Is your Q-angle in this normal range? What anatomical factors may affect Q-angle?

6. Find a scientific peer-reviewed article that was published in the previous 5 years in which Q-angle was assessed. In your own words, what was the purpose of that study, why was Q-angle assessed, and were significant differences (in terms of Q-angle) reported in that study? Copy the abstract and include it at the end of this laboratory assignment.

7. In the last column of the measurement sheet, calculate the active ROM for the subject's left and right knees. Active ROM = active knee flexion angle – active knee extension angle.

8. In the last column of the measurement sheet, calculate the passive ROM for the subject's left and right knees. Passive ROM = passive knee flexion angle – passive knee extension angle.

9. Compare the subject's active and passive knee ROM for the left and right legs. Which is greater, active or passive ROM? Why?

210   Unit Three Laboratories

Isokinetic Strength Assessment Laboratory

Objective of this lab: The purpose of this lab is to provide students with hands-on experience in participating in an isokinetic strength assessment as well as processing isokinetic strength data in Excel.

Key Concepts:

1. Students will be the "subject" or a "tester" in an isokinetic strength assessment.

2. Using Microsoft Excel, students will process data of an isokinetic strength assessment. Namely, knee extension and flexion peak torque, peak torque normalized to body weight, average torque, and joint power will be calculated, as well as the hamstring/quadriceps ratio.

3. Students will use a search engine such as PubMed to find a peer-reviewed scientific research article dealing with isokinetic strength assessment. Students will also interpret results of this research article.

Equipment:

Biodex System 4 Isokinetic Dynamometer

Attire:

Students will arrive at the laboratory session in a short-sleeve T-shirt, shorts, and athletic shoes.

Procedures:

1. Students will divide into groups of 3. Each group will select a " subject." The others in the group will be "testers."

2. The subject will be seated in the Biodex chair. The testers adjust the position of the Biodex chair so that the subject's knee is aligned with the axis of the dynamometer. They will then strap the subject's lower leg onto the arm of the dynamometer.

3. The course instructor will create a new "Patient" file on the computer for the subject. The subject will provide his or her body weight.

> Body weight in pounds: _____ → Body mass in kg: _____
>
> Conversion factor: Body mass in kg = Body weight in pounds / 2.2

4. The testers will set the range of motion of the leg, align the lower leg with vertical, and weigh the leg.

5. Five trials of knee extension and flexion will then be collected at 60 degrees/second. These will be saved for future analysis. These data files will be uploaded onto SOLE by the end of the day.

6. Steps 2–5 will be repeated until each group has performed the lab.

Unit Three Laboratories   211

Data Processing:

1. Open Microsoft Excel™. All data processing will be done in Microsoft Excel.

2. Open the data file in Excel. It should look similar to the following, but much longer.

TIME mSec	TORQUE N-M	POS (ANAT) Degrees	VELOCITY DEG/SEC
0	0	102	−0.2
10	0.5	102	0.7
20	0.5	102	0.5
30	0.7	102	0.2
40	0.5	102	0.7
50	3.5	102	1.8
60	3.5	102	1.5
70	3.5	102	2.1
80	3.5	102	2.3
90	3.4	102	2.9
100	3.4	102	3.4
110	2.8	102	3.4

3. Notice the following:

   a. Column 1 = Time (msec)

   b. Column 2 = Torque (Nm)

   c. Column 3 = Anatomical Position (degrees)

   d. Column 4 = Velocity (degrees/sec)

4. Plot each of the following using the "Scattergraph" function. (Go to the Insert tab at the top of the page, click on "Scatter," and select the type of graph you wish to use.) Note: You may highlight non-adjacent columns in Excel by holding down the <Ctrl> key when you click on the column.

   Plot:

   a. Time vs. Torque

   b. Time vs. Position

   c. Time vs. Velocity

   Make sure that each graph has a title, x-axis label, and y-axis label. Include the appropriate units in the labels of the axes. DO NOT include a legend on each graph because there will only be one line on each graph; therefore, a legend is not necessary. An example of each graph with proper titles and axis labels is as follows:

212   Unit Three Laboratories

5. You will notice that there are five peaks and five valleys on the Time vs. Torque graph. The positive values represent the values for knee extension torque and the negative valleys represent the values for knee flexion torque.

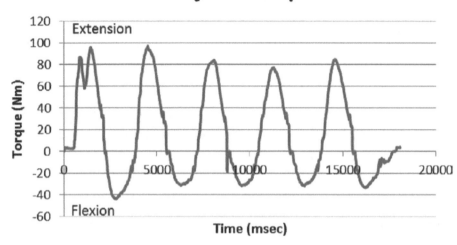

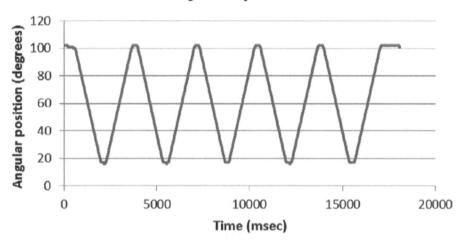

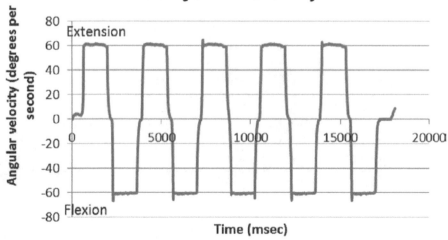

Unit Three Laboratories 213

Knee Extension Peak Torque

a. Look on the data spreadsheet (NOT on the graph) and find the positive peaks for knee extension. Record the values of these peaks in the "Knee Extension Peak Torque (Nm)" column in Table 1.

b. Divide each of these values by the subject's mass (in kg). Record these values in the "Knee Extension Peak Torque normalized to body mass (Nm/kg)" column in Table 1.

c. Calculate the average of each of these measurements and record these values in the final row of Table 1.

Table 1: Knee Extension Peak Torque Results

	Knee Extension Peak Torque (Nm)	Knee Extension Peak Torque Normalized to Body Mass (Nm/kg)
Trial 1		
Trial 2		
Trial 3		
Trial 4		
Trial 5		
Average		

d. Determine the knee joint angle (in degrees) at the time of knee extension peak torque. Record these values in Table 2.

Table 2: Angle of Knee Extension Peak Torque (Degrees)

	Knee Joint Angle at Knee Extension Peak Torque (Degrees)
Trial 1	
Trial 2	
Trial 3	
Trial 4	
Trial 5	
Average	

214 Unit Three Laboratories

Knee Flexion Peak Torque

a. Look on the data spreadsheet (NOT on the graph) and find the negative peaks for knee flexion. Record the values of these peaks in the "Knee Flexion Peak Torque (Nm)" column in Table 3.

b. Divide each of these values by the subject's mass (in kg). Record these values in the "Knee Flexion Peak Torque Normalized to Body Mass (Nm/kg)" column in Table 3.

c. Calculate the average of each of these measurements and record these values in the final row of Table 3.

Table 3: Knee Flexion Peak Torque Results

	Knee Flexion Peak Torque (Nm)	Knee Flexion Peak Torque Normalized to Body Mass (Nm/kg)
Trial 1		
Trial 2		
Trial 3		
Trial 4		
Trial 5		
Average		

d. Determine the knee joint angle (in degrees) at the time of knee flexion peak torque. Record these values in Table 4.

	Knee Joint Angle at Knee Flexion Peak Torque (Degrees)
Trial 1	
Trial 2	
Trial 3	
Trial 4	
Trial 5	
Average	

Unit Three Laboratories 215

6. Joint Power (and working with a formula in an Excel spreadsheet)

In linear terms, power equals force × velocity. In angular terms, power equals torque × angular velocity.

$$\text{Power} = \text{Torque} \times \text{Angular velocity}$$

The units for power are watts.

   a. In the Excel spreadsheet, make a fifth column and label it "Power."

   b. In the first data row of this column (this should be row 3), enter the following formula:

   $$= B3 * D3 \text{ (i.e., Knee torque} \times \text{knee angular velocity)}$$

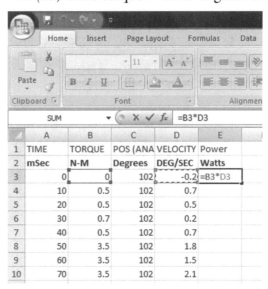

   c. Drag this formula down the entire column, so that your column appears similar to the one in the figure below.

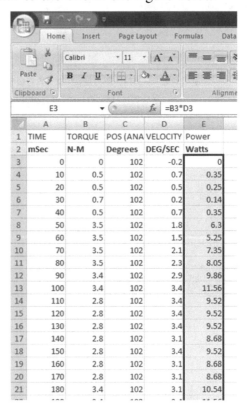

d. Plot the knee joint power, as shown in the example graph below.

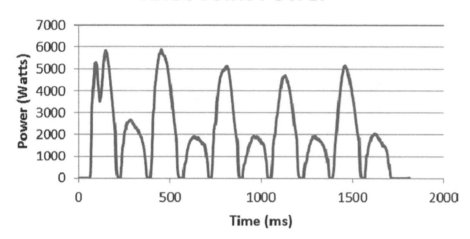

Questions

1. Look at the Time vs. Velocity graph. What was the average maximum angular velocity during knee extension? During knee flexion? How were these values determined? What does the "sign" on the angular velocity indicate?

2. Which was stronger, knee extension peak torque or knee flexion peak torque? Why do you think that is? (Hint: What determines muscle force? What determines joint torque?)

3. Calculate the knee joint flexion/extension ratio. (Average knee flexion peak torque/average knee extension peak torque.) At this velocity, the "ideal" value is 0.62. If your calculated value is not close to this number, hypothesize why this muscle imbalance exists.

4. What is the purpose of normalizing strength to body mass?

5. Does knee extension or knee flexion have greater power? Why?

6. Thus far, knee joint torque has been (+) for extension and (–) for flexion. Also, knee joint velocity has been (+) for extension and (–) for flexion. Why are almost all of the data points in the knee joint power column positive? Also, do you think this power represents concentric or eccentric power? Why?

7. Find a scientific peer-reviewed article that was published in the previous 5 years in which the isokinetic strength of the knee musculature was assessed. In your own words, what was the purpose of that study, why was strength assessed, and were significant differences (in terms of strength) reported in that study? Copy the abstract and include it at the end of this laboratory assignment.

Isokinetic Strength Assessment Laboratory Assignment

To be submitted on: _____ (date due)

Even though you collected data in a group, each student is required to submit an INDIVIDUAL lab report that contains the following items:

- The names of the other students in your group. (Even though you are submitting individual laboratory reports, we still want to know which of you will be using the same data files.)

- Using Microsoft Word, a typed copy of Tables 1–4. Use the "Table" function. Do not use tabs or spaces to create a table.

  - Table 1: Knee Extension Peak Torque

  - Table 2: Angle at Knee Extension Peak Torque

  - Table 3: Knee Flexion Peak Torque

  - Table 4: Angle at Knee Flexion Peak Torque

- The following graphs, made in Microsoft Excel. If desired, these may be pasted into Word or into a PDF for submission of the assignment.

  - Knee Joint Torque vs. Time

  - Knee Joint Position vs. Time

  - Knee Joint Velocity vs. Time

  - Knee Joint Power vs. Time

- The answers to questions 1–7. Note: Question 7 requires that you also submit an abstract of a research article in which the isokinetic strength of the knee musculature was assessed.

Unit Three Laboratories   221

Unit Four Laboratories

Name: _____

Resting and Exercise Heart Rates and Blood Pressure

Objective of this lab: To perform resting and exercising blood pressure and heart-rate measurements using auscultation and radial artery palpation.

Key Concepts:

1. Become proficient in the correct use of the blood pressure cuff and the stethoscope (e.g., choosing the correct size of cuff, correct placement of cuff and stethoscope on arm, correct placement of stethoscope in ears, inflation/deflation of cuff, etc.).

2. Ability to utilize techniques for augmenting auscultation of blood pressure.

3. Identify correct anatomical sites for heart-rate palpation.

Instructions

1. Each group needs to obtain two (2) stethoscopes and two (2) blood pressure cuffs.

2. Two members of each group will practice obtaining resting blood pressure and heart-rate measurements on the other two members of the group.

   a. Be sure to determine if it is safe to obtain a blood pressure in the arm you wish to measure.

3. Switch with other members in your group so that you are a subject and they become the test administrators.

4. Record three blood pressure and heart-rate measurements for each member of your group.

	Person 1	Person 2	Person 3
Name			
Blood pressure 1			
Heart rate 1			
Blood Pressure 2			
Heart rate 2			
Blood pressure 3			
Heart rate 3			

5. Be sure at least one of the above measurements is performed with the instructor observing and listening using a dual teaching stethoscope.

6. Have two members of each group walk on treadmills at a comfortable walking pace (2.0–3.0 mph).

7. Practice obtaining blood pressure and heart-rate measurements of those individuals walking on treadmills.

8. Switch with other members in your group so that you are a subject and they become the test administrators.

9. Record three exercising blood pressure and heart-rate measurements for each member of your group.

Exercising Blood Pressures

	Person 1	Person 2	Person 3
Name			
Blood pressure 1			
Heart rate 1			
Blood Pressure 2			
Heart rate 2			

10. Be sure at least one of the above measurements is performed with the instructor observing and listening using a dual teaching stethoscope.

11. After walking on the treadmill, sit and cool down for 5 minutes and repeat the heart-rate and blood pressure measurements.

    BP: _____ HR: _____

12. After completing the HR and BP measurements following 5 minutes of rest, perform push-up exercises until volitional fatigue. Obtain a BP and HR reading immediately upon completion of the push-up exercises.

    BP: _____ HR: _____

Questions

1. Classify (categorize) the resting blood pressure measurements of the individuals in your group (e.g., optimal/normal, prehypertensive, etc.).

2. What was the heart-rate and blood pressure (both systolic and diastolic) response of each individual to walking on the treadmill? Is this a normal or abnormal response? Explain.

3. What was the heart-rate and blood pressure (both systolic and diastolic) response of each individual to performing push-up exercises? Is this a normal or abnormal response? Explain. Compare this response to the response observed during treadmill walking.

4. What three things can you do to help ensure that you hear the Korotkoff sounds while taking a blood pressure?

5. List the other anatomical locations from which the arterial pulse can be obtained.

Unit Four Laboratories   225

Resting and Exercise ECGs

Objective of this lab: To administer and interpret resting and exercising ECGs.

Key Concepts:

1. Understand the correct anatomical locations for electrode placement for recording of the six limb leads.

2. Understand and identify factors that increase/decrease the artifact observed at rest and during exercise on an ECG tracing.

3. Understand how time and magnitude can be measured on standard ECG paper.

4. Ability to print and interpret ECG strips from the six limb leads.

5. Ability to correctly measure duration and magnitude of various waveforms and segments (e.g., P-R interval, QRS duration, S-T segment elevation and/or depression, etc.).

6. Understand how exercise can affect waveform morphology, duration, and magnitude.

7. Understand what a normal sinus rhythm looks like in the six limb leads.

Instructions

1. Identify the correct anatomical locations for electrode placement for obtaining a six-limb-lead ECG.

2. Shave the areas if needed.

3. Clean the areas with alcohol and gauze.

4. Apply electrodes to the subject and attach the ECG leads in their correct location.

5. Turn on the ECG monitor and verify no artifact is present at rest on the ECG tracing.

6. Record resting ECG strips for all six limb leads.

7. Secure ECG leads to person's waist using supplied belt.

8. Have subject walk on a treadmill for 5 minutes at 3.0 mph and 0% grade.

9. Record ECG strips for all six limb leads at the end of each minute during the treadmill walk.

Unit Four Laboratories   227

Questions

1. Label the P, Q, R, S, and T waves on all of your ECG recordings.

2. For all six of the limb leads, answer the following:

    a. Describe what the P wave looks like. What does the P wave represent in terms of what is occurring in the myocardium?

    b. Describe what the QRS complex looks like. What does the QRS complex represent in terms of what is occurring in the myocardium?

    c. Describe what the T wave looks like. What does the T wave represent in terms of what is occurring in the myocardium?

    d. Measure the P-R interval. Is the P-R interval within normal limits? What does the P-R interval represent in terms of what is occurring in the myocardium? What conditions are associated with an increased or decreased P-R interval?

    e. Measure the QRS interval. Is the QRS interval within normal limits? What does the QRS interval represent in terms of what is occurring in the myocardium? What conditions are associated with an increased or decreased QRS interval?

Unit Four Laboratories   229

f. Describe what the S-T segment looks like in all six limb leads at rest and during exercise (e.g., is the S-T segment horizontal, down sloping, up sloping, depressed, or elevated?) What conditions are associated with abnormal S-T segments?

3. Describe any differences between the resting and exercising ECG tracings.

4. List and explain sources of artifact on a resting and exercising ECG tracing.

Unit Five Laboratories

Name: _____

Spirometry

Objective of this lab: To understand the principles of spirometry, its clinical importance, and the methods used to measure lung volumes and capacities.

Key Concepts:

1. Measurements of lung volumes and forced expiratory flow rates are commonly used tests of lung function in clinical practice. They are easily performed and offer considerable diagnostic and prognostic value in many lung disorders. They often permit quantification of the functional disorder and allow progression or regression of disease to be followed objectively over time.

2. Two distinct patterns of disorder are most readily observed with data obtained from the flow-volume loop and volume-time graphs (see Table 1).

   Airflow obstruction (chronic airflow obstruction, e.g., chronic bronchitis, emphysema; reversible airflow obstruction, e.g., asthma). In these disorders maximal expiratory flow rates and vital capacity are reduced. In particular, the fraction of the forced vital capacity (FVC) that can be exhaled in the first second ($FEV_{1.0}$/FVC ratio) is reduced. Another common index of airflow obstruction is mean flow rate in the middle half of a forced vital capacity expiration (FEF_{25-75}). There is usually an increase in residual volume and functional residual capacity. Total lung capacity is typically increased.

   Restrictive lung disorders (e.g., fibrosing alveolitis, sarcoidosis). These disorders are characterized by reduced vital capacity, residual volume, functional residual capacity, and total lung capacity. $FEV_{1.0}$/FVC ratio and expiratory flow rates are normal or even increased relative to absolute lung volume.

3. Understand what volumes and/or capacities can be measured via simple spirometry and which cannot.

4. Understand the principals involved in using the oxygen dilution technique and the purpose for performing this test.

Instructions

1. Select a volunteer to have lung volume measurement taken.

2. Obtain and record test subject's age, height, and sex.

3. Obtain and record barometric pressure, temperature, and humidity.

4. With assistance from the instructor, perform a simple spirometry test.

5. With assistance from the instructor, perform a maximal voluntary ventilation (MVV) test.

6. With assistance from the instructor, perform the oxygen dilution test.

Unit Five Laboratories   231

TABLE 1

Typical Volume and Flow Rate Patterns

	Normal	Obstructive Disease	Restrictive Disease
TLC (ml)	7500	8000	5000
VC (ml)	6000	4000	4000
RV (ml)	1500	4000	1000
FVC (ml)	6000	3600	4000
$FEV_{1.0}$ (ml)	4800	1800	3500
$FEV_{1.0}$/FVC (%)	80%	50%	88%
FEF_{25-75}(L/sec)	4.0	1.0	3.6

OXYGEN DILUTION METHOD TO MEASURE RESIDUAL VOLUME

1. (Wilmore, J. H., Vodak, P. A.,&PARR, R. P., et al. (1980). Further simplification of a method for determination of residual lung volume. *Medicine & Science in Sports & Exercise*, 12(3), 216–218.) Turn on O_2/CO_2 analyzers (allow for 30 minutes to warm up before use).

2. Turn on laptop computer with OMI spirometer. Open OMI spirometer software.

3. Attach two-way breathing value to spirometer.

4. Flush the spirometer with 100% O_2.

   a. Close valve to spirometer, fill the spirometer with 100% O_2 (not more the 9 L)

   b. Open valve to air to allow the gas in spirometer to escape, close valve to spirometer before it is fully empty.

   c. Repeat steps 4a and 4btwice.

   d. On the last fill with O_2, fill spirometer half way (i.e. 4 to 5 L) with 100% O_2 and **leave valve closed to spirometer.**

5. **Measure** and **record** O_2 and CO_2 levels in the spirometer from sampling port.

6. **Record spirometer volume**.

   a. Go to Calibration Menu in OMI spirometer software

   b. Select Linearity check

   c. Click OK

   d. Read "Current Volume = xxxx mL"

7. Have a volunteer sit comfortably in front of spirometer with *clean* mouthpiece filter securely positioned on the two-way valve.

   a. Instruct volunteer to place on nose clips.

   b. Have the volunteer get comfortable on the mouthpiece (*valve is still closed to spirometer,* the subject is simply breathing room air through the valve).

   c. Have the volunteer exhale to RV, *when reaching RV open valve to the spirometer* quickly allowing subject to breath in from the spirometer.

   d. Have the subject take seven deep breaths at rate of 1 breath every 2 seconds. **The rate and depth of breathing is critical for efficient mixing of gas between the lung and spirometer!**

   e. After the end of the 7th breath, immediately turn valve closed to the spirometer and the subject can come off the mouthpiece.

8. **Measure** and **record** final O_2 and CO_2 levels in the spirometer from sampling port (*ensure stable reading before recording O_2/CO_2 values, i.e. sample for at least 30 seconds*).

Initial $O_2\%$ (O_{2i})	Initial $CO_2\%$ (CO_{2i})	Initial Volume (Vi), L	Final $O_2\%$ (O_{2f})	Final $CO_2\%$ (CO_{2f})

9. Use the following equation to calculate RV: $\mathbf{RV = Vi \times (b - a)/(c - d)}$

   where,

   a = % of N_2 at the initial volume, i.e. a = $100 - (O_{2i} + CO_{2i})$;

   a = _____

   b = % of N_2 after gas mixing between lung and spirometer, i.e. $100 - (O_{2f} + CO_{2f})$;

   b = _____

   c = % of N_2 in alveolar air at beginning of test (assumed to be 79);

   c = _____

   d = % of N_2 in alveolar air during last breath (assumed to be 0.2% N_2 than b, i.e. b + 0.2%);

   d = _____

Once you have calculated RV, you need to subtract deadspace volume of the *airways* (= 1 mL for each pound of lean body mass) and the *device* (= 200 mL). RV = Calculated RV – Air dead space = Device dead space

Remember: RV is approximately 20 to 25% of FVC. How close is your estimated RV compared to your measured RV?

Questions

1. Draw a normal spirogram and label the subdivisions of the vital capacity.

2. What lung volumes are not accessible to direct measurement with a spirometer? Name two methods for measuring these volumes.

3. Which airways contribute most to airway resistance in normal subjects?

4. What are the determinants of maximum expiratory flow after about the first 25% of a forced expiratory maneuver? Explain why flow rate is "effort independent" beyond this point.

5. What information is gain from performing the MVV test?

6. The oxygen dilution technique is used to measure what lung volumes or capacities. Calculate the "measured volume" using the values given in the lab.

7. **Remember:** RV is approximately 20–25% of FVC. How close is your estimated RV compared to your measured RV?

Unit 1

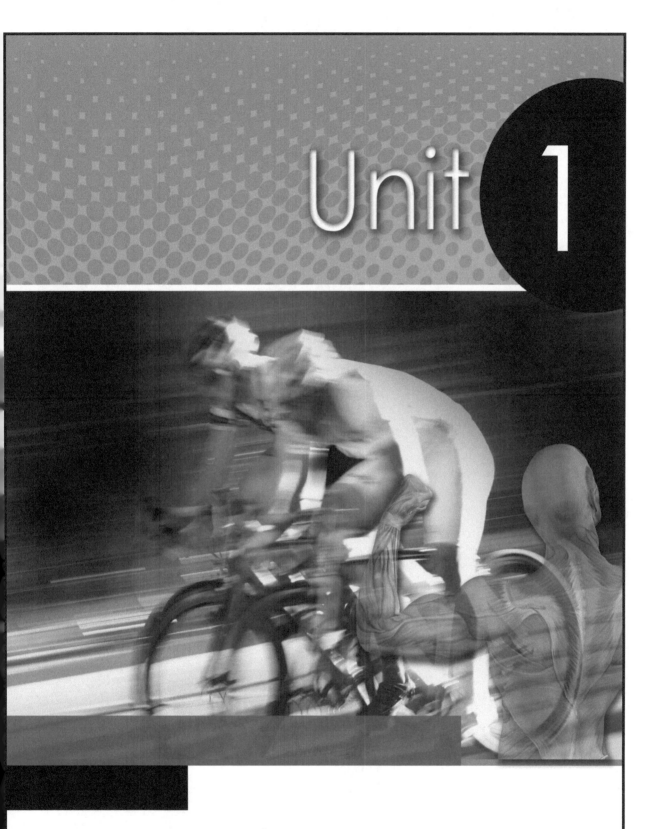

Exercise and the Endocrine System

13

Exercise and the Endocrine System

The endocrine system, along with the nervous system, regulates all of homeostasis, integrating body functions in order to provide a stable internal environment.

AFFECT NEARLY ALL ASPECTS OF HUMAN FUNCTION:

- Activate enzymes
- Alter cell membrane permeability
- Initiate muscle contraction and relaxation
- Stimulate protein and fat synthesis
- Cause cellular secretion
- Respond to stress

The endocrine system is relatively small compared with other organs.

ENDOCRINE ORGANS:

- Pineal gland
- Hypothalamus (considered the neuroendocrine organ)
- Pituitary gland
- Thyroid gland
- Parathyroid glands
- Thymus gland
- Adrenal gland
- Pancreas

- Gonads (sex organs—ovary, testes)
- Adipose tissue

Consists of *gland* (host organ), *hormones* (chemical messengers), and *target/receptor organ*.

Glands are classified as either **endocrine** or **exocrine.**

CHARACTERISTICS OF THE ENDOCRINE SYSTEM

No ducts (ductless glands)

Secrete substances into extracellular spaces

Diffuses into bloodstream for transport to target tissues in the body

CHARACTERISTICS OF THE EXOCRINE SYSTEM

Contain secretory ducts

Able to carry substances directly to surface or compartment

Primary control via nervous system

Examples: sweat glands and upper GI glands

Definition of a hormone: chemical substances synthesized by glands, secreted into the blood, and carried throughout the body.

Types of Hormones

Two chemical categories of hormones:

1. Steroid-derived hormones: not soluble in blood plasma; synthesized from circulating *cholesterol* via adrenal cortex and gonads; receptors are usually found *within* the cell.

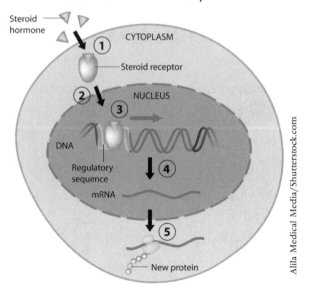

2. Hormones synthesized from amino acids (amine or polypeptide hormones): soluble in blood plasma; receptors are located on the *cell membrane* of target tissues.

MECHANISMS OF HORMONE ACTION

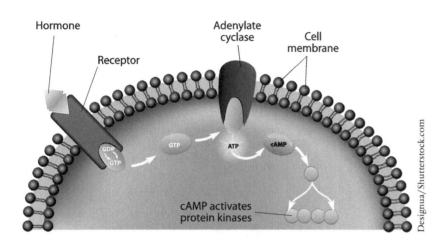

Hormone/Target Cell Specificity

Major Function:

To alter the rates of cellular reactions of specific target cells by:

1. modifying rate of intracellular protein synthesis via DNA stimulation;
2. changing rate of enzyme activity;
3. altering plasma membrane transport via second messenger; and
4. Inducing secretory activity.

Target cell's ability to respond to a hormone depends on the presence of specific protein receptors that bind the hormone in a complementary way.

Target cell receptors occur in either of the following ways:

Hormone-receptor binding is the first step in initiating hormonal action.

Target cell's activation by hormone depends on *three* factors:

1.
2.
3.

Cell hormone receptors are dynamic and constantly adjust to physiologic demands:

Up-regulation: target cells form more receptors in response to increasing hormone levels.

Down-regulation: a loss of receptor which prevents target cells from overresponding to persistently high hormone levels (desensitizes target cells).

Cyclic AMP:

Which hormone has its receptor in the cell membrane? How does it get its message inside?

An intracellular messenger produced from the binding hormone (first messenger) reacting to the enzyme adenylate cyclase (plasma membrane) forming cyclic 3′5′-adenosine monophosphate (cyclic AMP) from an original ATP.

Cyclic AMP becomes second messenger and activates a specific protein kinase, which then activates a target enzyme to alter cellular function, which is the ultimate goal.

Altering enzyme activity and enzyme-mediated membrane transport are major hormone actions.

Hormones increase enzyme activity in one of three ways:

1. Stimulating enzyme production;

2. Combining with the enzyme to alter its shape and ability to act (allosteric modulation), which can either increase or decrease the enzyme catalytic effectiveness;

3. Activating inactive forms of the enzyme, increasing total amount of active enzyme.

Factors That Determine Hormone Levels:

How often is the hormone released or secreted? Secretion rarely occurs at a constant rate.

Secretion rate is adjusted rapidly to meet the demands of changing bodily conditions.

Secretory patterns differ among hormones. All protein hormones secrete in a pulsatile manner.

The actual plasma concentration of a hormone depends on four factors:

1. Amount synthesized in the host gland

2. Rate of either catabolism or secretion into the blood.

3. Quantity of transport proteins available.

4. Plasma volume changes.

Endocrine glands are stimulated by one of three methods:

Hormonal Stimulation:

• Many hormones influence the secretion of other hormones (many times in the form of negative feedback loop). What is a tropic hormone?

Humeral Stimulation:

• Changing levels of certain ions and nutrients in blood, bile, and other body fluids also stimulate hormone release

242   Chapter 13—Exercise and the Endocrine System

Neural Stimulation:

- Hormone release is also affected by neural activity (e.g., sympathetic nervous system releases norepinephrine and epinephrine during periods of stress)

Anterior Pituitary Hormones

Pituitary gland (hypophysis)

- Often referred to as the master gland;
- Located beneath base of brain;
- Secretes at least six different peptide hormones;
- Controlled by **hypothalamus**, which secretes *releasing factors* for each of the primary hormones released from the anterior pituitary.

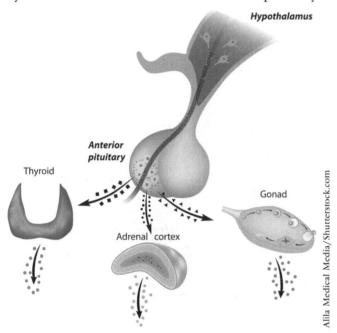

Growth Hormone (GH)

Growth hormone-releasing factor from hypothalamus directly stimulates the anterior pituitary gland for the secretion of GH.

GH secretion occurs throughout life.

GH exerts widespread physiologic activity by:

1. Promoting cell division and proliferation.
    A. Affects all aspects of cartilage growth
    B. Increases linear bone growth
    C. Increases width of bones
2. Increasing protein synthesis in adult cells by increasing amino acid transport across cell membrane, stimulating RNA formation, and activating cellular ribosomes.
3. Decreasing in CHO breakdown and an increase in the mobilization of lipids as energy.

GH is stimulated by hypoglycemia, fasting, starvation, increased blood amino acid levels, and stress (trauma, excitement, emotional, and ***heavy exercise***).

GH is stimulated by an acute bout of exercise (increases pulse amplitude) and is dependent on exercise intensity and duration.

Appears to stimulate isoforms that have longer half-life

Augments protein synthesis

Also decreases tissue glucose uptake, increasing free fatty acid mobilization, and enhances liver glucogenogenesis.

Both fit and sedentary individuals show similar increases in GH when exercising to exhaustion; sedentary individuals show greater response during submaximal exercise and into recovery.

Cause of release during exercise is not known:

- Direct stimulatory affect
- May stimulate cholinergic pathways to cause release
- May work through endogenous opioids
- May involve elevations in core body temperature

Insulin-like Growth Factors (IGF):

- Mediate many of GH's effects
- Liver cells synthesize IGF-I and IGF-II in response to GH stimulation (usually 8 to 30 hours after GH release).

Thyrotropin (Thyroid-Stimulating Hormone [TSH])

Controls amount of hormone secretion by the thyroid gland

Increases thyroid cell metabolism and acts to maintain growth and development of the thyroid gland

Increase in TSH does not occur consistently in response to exercise

Adrenocorticotropic Hormone (Corticotropin)

Adrenocorticotropic hormone (ACTH) functions as part of the hypothalamic-pituitary–adrenal axis and regulates output of hormones secreted by the adrenal cortex in a manner similar to TSH control of thyroid gland secretion.

ACTH acts directly to:

-
-
-

Release of ACTH is controlled by corticotropin-releasing hormone (CRH) and arginine vasopressin (AVP).

CRH is released during periods of fever, hypoglycemia, and other stressors.

Limited data has indicated that ACTH concentrations may increase proportionally with exercise intensity and duration.

244   Chapter 13—Exercise and the Endocrine System

Prolactin

Initiates and supports milk secretion from mammary glands

Increases at high exercise intensities and recovers toward baseline within 45 minutes

Repeated exercise-induced prolactin release may alter menstrual cycle

Gonadotropic Hormones

Stimulate male and female sex organs to grow and secrete their hormones at a faster rate.

- Follicle-stimulating hormone (FSH): initiates growth in the ovaries and stimulates them to secrete estrogen. In males, aids in sperm development.

- Luteinizing hormone (LH): complement of FSH causing estrogen secretion and rupture of follicle. In males, stimulates testes to secrete testosterone.

Although difficult to measure because of the pulsatile nature of release, limited data indicate that *acute* exercise may stimulate release (especially LH).

However, *chronic high-intensity aerobic training* has been reported to decrease the pulse amplitude and frequency of the gonadotropic hormones.

Additional Hormones:

Endogenous Opioids

- Strongly inhibit LH and FSH release from AP

- Stimulate GH and prolactin release

- Released during exercise

- May be associated with increase pain tolerance, improved appetite control, reduced anxiety, tension, anger and confusion

Posterior Pituitary Hormones

Posterior pituitary is an outgrowth of the hypothalamus.

Hormones secreted from the posterior pituitary are actually made in the hypothalamus and then secreted into the posterior pituitary to be stored until needed (two specifically):

1. Antidiuretic hormone (ADH or vasopressin) influences water excretion by the kidneys by stimulating reabsorption thus decreasing urine output.

2. Oxytocin initiates muscle contraction in the uterus and stimulates ejection of milk.

Exercise is an important stimulant for ADH secretion and release.

Thyroid Hormones

The thyroid is located in the neck just below larynx.

The thyroid is under the control of TSH that is secreted from pituitary gland.

Chapter 13—Exercise and the Endocrine System   245

The thyroid secretes two protein–iodine-bound hormones:

1. **Thyroxine** (T_4): converted to T_3 by most receptor cells. This hormone raises the metabolism of all cells except brain, spleen, testes, uterus, and thyroid itself. Abnormal increase raises basal metabolic rate (BMR) up to four times; hyposecretion would result in the opposite.

2. **Triiodothyronine** (T_3): acts faster than T_4 but is secreted in less quantity than T_4.

Thyroid hormones also provide important regulation for tissue growth and development, skeletal and nervous system formation, and maturation and reproductive capabilities.

Thyroid hormones also play a role in maintaining blood pressure by causing an increase in adrenergic receptors in blood vessels.

During exercise, blood levels of free T_4 increase by approximately 35% (possibly caused by elevated core body temperature).

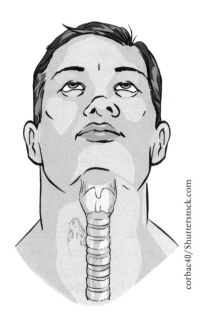

Parathyroid Hormone (PTH)

The parathyroid gland is made of four small glands embedded in the posterior aspect of the thyroid gland.

PTH controls blood calcium balance.

Release of PTH is triggered by decrease in blood calcium levels and is inhibited by increasing levels.

PTH stimulates three target organs: bone, kidney, and small intestine.

Physical activity may increase PTH, an effect that may contribute to the positive effects of exercise on bone mass.

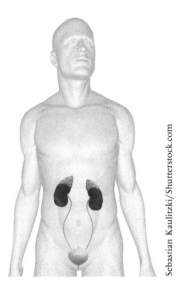

Adrenal Medulla Hormones

The adrenal medulla is part of sympathetic nervous system.

The adrenal medulla works to prolong sympathetic effects by secreting two hormones collectively called catecholamines:

Epinephrine and Norepinephrine:

Norepinephrine serves as epinephrine precursor and also acts as a neurotransmitter when released by sympathetic nerve endings.

Nerve impulses from the hypothalamus stimulate adrenal medulla to increase these hormones.

Epinephrine's major effects on the heart, blood vessels, and glands are similar to those of the sympathetic nervous system *except slower*.

Additional functions include:

- Epinephrine stimulates glycogenolysis (primarily liver) and lipolysis (adipose and muscle)
- Norepinephrine stimulates lipolysis in the adipose tissue

Both increase with exercise, and are **related to intensity**.

Athletes involved in sprint-power training show greater sympathoadrenergic activation during maximal exercise than aerobically-trained athletes.

Activation of the adrenal medulla and its effects on blood flow distribution, cardiac contractility, and energy substrate mobilization all benefit the exercise response.

How does exercise intensity affect release? Draw the relationship.

Chapter 13—Exercise and the Endocrine System

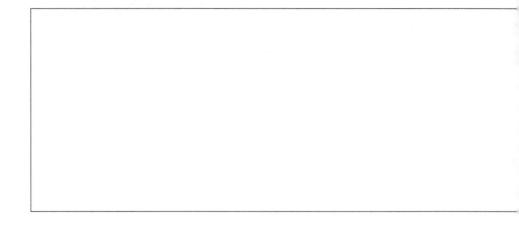

ADRENOCORTICAL HORMONES:

Secreted by the adrenal cortex

Categorized into three groups:

1. Mineralocorticoids:

    Regulate the mineral salts such as Na^+ and K^+ in the extracellular fluid spaces.

    Aldosterone is the most important (95% of all mineralocorticoids are aldosterone).

    - Control total Na^+ concentration as well as extracellular fluid volume.
    - Regulate sodium reabsorption in the distal tubules of the kidneys.
    - For every Na reabsorbed, K and/or H are exchanged, which helps control proper mineral balance.

    Increases in aldosterone:

    - Cause Na reabsorption resulting in little Na fluid voided in urine.
    - Cause an increase in cardiac output and increase in BP (renin–angiotensin mechanism).

    Decrease in aldosterone causes decrease in Na and water reabsorption

    Cellular responses to aldosterone are slow

    It requires relatively prolonged exercise (>45 min) for aldosterone's effect to emerge (usually see affect during recovery)

2. Glucocorticoids:

    Are ideally suited for severe stress situations.

    Hypothalamus will release corticotropin-releasing factor causing anterior pituitary to release ACTH which promotes release of glucocorticoids by adrenal cortex.

    Cortisol is the major glucocorticoid, and affects glucose, protein, and free fatty acid metabolism.

    Why would cortisol increase during exercise?

3. Gonadocorticoids:

Androgen hormones with similar actions as certain sex steroids produced from the reproductive organs (i.e., testosterone).

Produce primarily *DHEA* (dehyroepiandrosterone), which has effects similar to male testosterone.

Also produce small amounts of estrogen and progesterone.

Gonadal Hormones

Reproductive glands:

Testes (male) and ovaries (female).

There are no distinct male and female hormones, but there are general differences in hormone concentrations between the sexes.

1. Testosterone

    Initiates sperm production and male secondary sex characteristics. Also has an anabolic/ tissue-building role.

    Promotes GH release and therefore IGF (indirect effect).

    Interacts with neural receptors to increase neurotransmitter release; alters size of neuromuscular junction.

    In untrained males, both resistance exercise and moderate aerobic exercise increase serum and free levels after 15 to 20 minutes.

    Values may remain elevated for at least 1 hour post strenuous exercise

2. Estrogens (estradiol and progesterone)

    Regulates ovulation, menstruation, and physiologic adjustments during pregnancy.

    Also plays an important role in bone development and health.

Hormonal Disturbances

Women who train intensely and emphasize weight loss often engage in disordered eating behaviors.

High levels of training and aberrant eating behaviors often decrease energy availability, reducing body mass and body fat to a point that:

1. creates irregularities in menstrual cycle function (*oligomenorrhea*; 35 to 90 days between periods)

2. causes cessation of menstruation (*secondary amenorrhea*)

Female Triad

Describes the coexistence of three distinct medical conditions that may occur in athletic girls and women.

Includes:

- Eating disorders/disordered eating behavior

- Amenorrhea/oligomenorrhea

- Decreased bone mineral density (osteoporosis and osteopenia)

Based on informal survey data, disordered eating behaviors occur in 15 to 60% of female athletes.

The prevalence of amenorrhea among female athletes in body weight-related sports (distance running, gymnastics, ballet, cheerleading, figure skating, body building) ranges between 25 and 65% (versus approximately 5% in the general population).

Cessation of menstruation removes estrogen's protective effect on bone, making these young women more vulnerable to injuries of the bone.

Estrogen's role in bone metabolism:

- Increases intestinal calcium absorption
- Reduces urinary calcium excretion
- Inhibits bone resorption
- Decreases bone turnover

Lowered bone density from extended amenorrhea often occurs at multiple sites, including bone areas subjected to increased force and impact loading during exercise.

This blunts the benefits of exercise on bone mass.

It increases the risk of musculoskeletal injuries, particularly repeated stress fractures during exercise.

Importance:

Bone mass may remain *permanently* at suboptimal levels throughout adult life— leaving the women at increased risk for osteoporosis and stress fractures.

The ACSM recommends that intervention begins within three months of the onset of amenorrhea.

Recommendations:

- Reduce training level by 10 to 20%
- Gradually increase total energy intake
- Increase body weight by 2 to 3%
- Maintain daily calcium intake at 1500 mg

Pancreatic Hormones

Pancreas gland is just below the stomach.

Pancreas is composed of two different types of tissues:

1. Acini (exocrine function):
2. Islets of Langerhans (endocrine cells):

    Contain alpha cells that secrete **glucagon** and beta cells that secrete **insulin**

Glucagon

Termed as "insulin antagonist."

Main function is to stimulate glycogenolysis and gluconeogenesis by the liver

Glucose released by this process is then released into the blood.

Glucagon is regulated by the amount of glucose in the blood.

Insulin

Major function is to regulate glucose entry into all tissues except the brain. Without this substance, only trace amounts of glucose can be transported into the cells.

Insulin regulates glucose metabolism.

Secretion is directly controlled by the level of glucose in the blood that passes through the pancreas.

Secretion is stimulated by increase in blood glucose levels.

Glucose Transport into Cells:

Insulin production increases the rate of glucose transport by promoting insertion of more glucose transport proteins (GLUT) into plasma membrane.

Muscle and adipose possess both non-insulin (GLUT-1) and insulin-mediated (GLUT-4) glucose uptake transporters.

Resting muscle: Most glucose enters the cell by a GLUT-1 carrier, which is responsible for low-level basal glucose uptake to sustain energy generation by cells. Can increase by fasting and decrease by excess amount of glucose.

When glucose and insulin levels are high or during exercise, most glucose enters muscle by (GLUT-4) transporter.

GLUT-4 is expressed exclusively in cardiac and skeletal muscle and adipose tissue.

GLUT-4 is specifically responsible for glucose utilization that is stimulated by insulin.

Exercise increases peripheral clearance in the presence of insulin through an insulin-dependent (an increased skeletal muscle insulin action) and an insulin-independent mechanism.

The increase in insulin action is associated with an increase in GLUT-4 and enzymes that regulate the storage and oxidation of glucose in skeletal muscle.

During rest, GLUT-4 resides near T-tubules of the SR.

When there is an influx of ions such as Na^+ or Ca^{2+}, the GLUT-4 transporter relocates to the cell surface through a separate insulin-independent mechanism to promote glucose uptake.

Effect of Insulin on Glucose Uptake

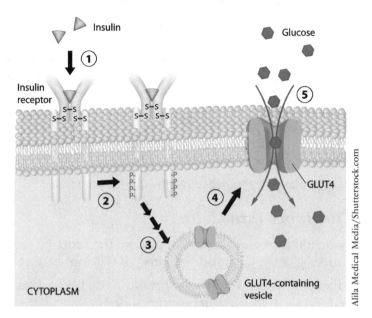

During exercise, insulin levels **decrease** significantly most likely due to epinephrine, which suppresses insulin secretion.

Levels of insulin **decrease** as a function of exercise duration **and** intensity.

Importance:

a. Takes away inhibitory effects of insulin on glucose production from gluconeogenesis (liver)

b. Minimizes glucose uptake by inactive tissues

c. With prolonged exercise, glucose and insulin decrease which enhances lipolysis and FFA availability.

d. In **trained** individuals, insulin does not fall as far as in untrained

Diabetes Mellitus

Some facts:

- Data from the 2011 National Diabetes Fact Sheet (released January 26, 2011
- Total: 25.8 million children and adults in the United States—8.3% of the population—have diabetes.
- Diagnosed: 18.8 million people
- Undiagnosed: 7.0 million people
- Prediabetic: 79 million people

Complications:

- At least 40% of cardiac patients have diabetes
- Sixth leading cause of death by disease
- Leading cause of adult blindness in the US

- Leading cause of non-traumatic amputation
- Leading cause of kidney disease in the US

Diagnosis criteria:

Random blood glucose of $\geq$ 200mg/dL

Fasting blood glucose of $\geq$ 126 mg/dL on two different occasions

Impaired fasting glucose of $\geq$110 to 125 mg/dL

Oral glucose tolerance test:

- Glucose is made to drink and two hours later glucose readings are taken
- If >200 mg/dL = positive
- If >140 mg/dL but < 200 mg/dL= impaired glucose tolerance

Definition: syndrome characterized by hyperglycemia resulting from impaired insulin secretion and/or effectiveness.

Type 1 Diabetes:

Usually occurs younger in life and represents 5 to 10% of all diabetes cases.

Characterized by an absolute deficiency of insulin and often other pancreatic hormones resulting from an autoimmune response (beta cells incapable of producing insulin).

More severe than type 2 for glucose homeostasis.

Effects of exercise on metabolic state are more pronounced—requires greater attention

- primarily concerned about hypoglycemia

Type 2 Diabetes:

Tends to occur after age 40 except in overweight children.

Accounts for 90% of the 16 million cases of diabetes.

Related to three factors:

1. The body's inability to respond properly to insulin's actions
2. An abnormal but relatively well-maintained insulin secretion (to a point)
3. Increased hepatic glucose production

Receptors or **post-receptor mechanisms** appear to be the problem due to the near normal to high levels of insulin present.

Therefore, not enough glucose will enter the cell, which in turn causes a high blood glucose level—very dangerous.

These patients are *insulin resistant*: body has overproduction of insulin in response to increased blood glucose of simple CHOs and sugars. This causes more glucose conversion and storage as body fat.

Chapter 13—Exercise and the Endocrine System   253

In association with insulin resistance, the glycolytic and oxidative capacities of the skeletal muscle are negatively affected.

The disease is most likely caused by genetic and lifestyle factors (i.e., physical inactivity, weight gain)

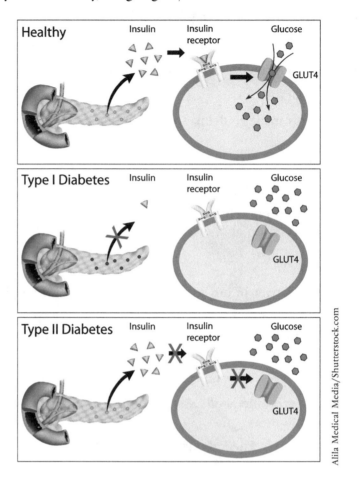

Physical Activity and Type 2 Diabetes:

Regular physical activity greatly reduces the risk of developing Type 2 diabetes

Benefits:

- Glycemic control: decreased plasma glucose levels
- Cardiovascular disease: reduced CAD risk
- Weight loss: decreased body fat enhances glucose tolerance and insulin sensitivity
- Psychological profile: decreased anxiety, improved mood and self-esteem
- Type 2 occurrence: delayed onset and even prevention for those at high risk for diabetes

What are the potential problems of exercising with type 2 diabetes?

Overview of Characteristics of Type 1 and 2 Diabetes

Characteristics	Type 1	Type 2
Age at onset	Usually <20 yrs	Usually >40 yrs
Proportion	<10%	>90%
Appearance of symptoms	Acute or subacute	Slow
Metabolic Ketoacidosis	Frequent	Rare
Obesity at onset	Uncommon	Common
B-cells	Decreased	Variable
Insulin	Decreased	Variable
Inflammatory islet cells	Present initially	Absent
Family history	Possibly	Common

Exercise and the Immune System

Natural immunity—also called *native* or *innate resistance,* is not produced by the immune response.

Acquired immunity—is gained after birth as a result of the immune response

Parts of the natural immune system:

    a.   Physical barriers

    b.   Chemical barriers

    c.   Certain cells

Parts of the acquired immune system:

    a.   Humoral

    b.   Cell-mediated

Circulating Leukocytes and Lymphocytes

Cell	% of Circulating Leukocytes	Primary Function
Granulocyte	60–70	
a. Neutrophil	> 90 of granulocytes	Phagocytosis
b. Eosinophil	2–5 of granulocytes	Phagocytosis of parasites
c. Basophil	0.2 of granulocytes	Chemotactic factor production
		Allergic response
Monocyte	10–15	Phagocytosis
		Antigen presentation
		Cytokine production
		Cytotoxicity
Lymphocyte	20–25	Lymphocyte activation
		Lymphokine production
		Antigen recognition
		Antibody production
		Memory
		Cytotoxicity

Cell	Percent of lymphocytes	Function
T cell		
a. T_H (CD4)		
b. T_C/T_{Ss}		
B cell		
LGL/NK		

256   Chapter 13—Exercise and the Endocrine System

CELL-MEDIATED IMMUNE RESPONSE

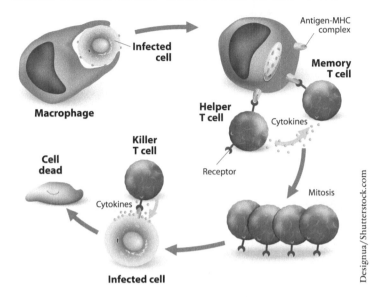

Leukocytosis (increase in circulating leukocyte number) is one of the most striking and consistent changes observed during exercise.

The magnitude of increases varies and is determined by a combination of exercise intensity and duration.

Exercise affects immune cell recirculation by altering the expression of cell adhesion molecules which is essential for their migration from tissues.

Granulocyte number increases markedly after strenuous or prolonged exercise but may not change after brief or low-intensity exercise.

In general, **moderate acute exercise** boosts neutrophil functions, including chemotaxis, phagocytosis, and oxidative burst activity. **Maximal exercise** appears to reduce these functions, with the exception of chemotaxis.

Lymphocytosis occurs during and immediately after exercise under a variety of conditions, from 10 min of stair climbing to marathon running. The magnitude of increase in lymphocyte number is generally **less** than for granulocytes and is related to exercise intensity. (Duration may not be important.)

Training may lessen the exercise induced response.

Unlike leukocyte or neutrophil numbers, lymphocyte numbers may **decrease** below resting levels before returning to normal after endurance exercise. (Exercise lasting 1 hour or more of relative high intensity/ > 70% VO_2max)

- Prolonged **acute** exercise is associated with a decrease in T-cell IL-2 and IFN-γ production immediately after exercise, and a decline in the number of circulating T cells that secrete IFN-γ. (*Reflects a decrease primarily of TH1 cells.*)

Following heavy exercise, there is an impairment of lymphocyte function as assessed in in vitro assays.

Mechanisms Underlying Changes in Leukocyte Distribution:

There is strong evidence that stress hormones act as mediators of exercise-induced changes in leukocyte number and subset redistribution.

Leukocytosis occurring during exercise has been simulated by exogenous administration of **epinephrin**e at appropriate concentrations seen with exercise and has been abrogated by beta-adrenergic blockade during exercise (Beta adrenoceptors have been shown to be present on natural killer (NK) T, and B cells, macrophages; and neutophils)

Corticosteroids given intravenously to humans cause lymphocytopenia, mono-cytopenia, eosinopenia, and neutrophilia which reach maximum 4 hours after administration.

Catecholamines and cortisol can both be immunosuppresive if chronically elevated.

Cytotoxic Cells:

Total NK activity is generally increased during and immediately after exercise whether brief or prolonged, moderate or intense.

For brief exercise (<30 min), NK activity is restored to resting levels by 1 hour after exercise.

In contract, maximal or prolonged exercise may **decrease** total activity for 1 to 6 hours after cessation of exercise.

Most data suggest that baseline NK activity is either unchanged or slightly **increased** by exercise **training**.

Conclusions (Training Effects):

Of all immune measures, only the NK cells has emerged as a somewhat **consistent** indicator differentiating the immune systems of athletes and non-athlete with NK cell activity being much higher in the athlete.

T cells which tend to function poorly in the elderly may perform at a higher level in **very fit** elderly individuals.

Antibodies

Antibody is an important effector of host resistance to infectious agents, and production of antibody is a major feature of the acquired immunity.

Immunoglobulins (Ig) are glycoproteins produced and secreted by B and plasma cells.

An antibody is an Ig molecule that reacts with a specific antigen.

The available data suggests that intense exercise does not by itself alter serum Ig and may increase specific antibodies.

However, the combination of intense training and psychological stress of competition may alter (lower) both total Ig and specific antibody levels.

In exercise-induced decreases in salivary and nasal wash, IgA levels have been reported in a variety of competitive athletes. It appears that the **cumulative** effects of intense daily training may have a more pronounced effect on IgA levels than a single exercise session.

Factors which can affect salivary IgA concentrations:

a. Intensity of the exercise session

b. The preceding training period

c. Psychological stress associated with training and competing at the elite level.

There does appear to be a temporal relationship between exercise-induced decreases in salivary IgA concentration and the appearance of URI.

However, moderate exercise training has been shown to restore optimal antibody in the face of stressors and ageing.

Risk of URS/URTI

"J"-shaped model of relationship between varying amounts of exercise and risk of URS/URTI. This model suggests that moderate exercise may lower risk of respiratory infection while excessive amounts may increase the risk.

Chronic Effect of Acute or Repeated Bouts of Exercise:

During a brisk walk, cells are recruited from the spleen, lungs, and other peripheral lymphoid tissues. They go into circulation and stay at an elevated level for approximately one to three hours post exercise before returning to normal.

During a brisk walk, there is no increase in stress hormones (e.g., cortisol and epinephrine) or proinflammatory cytokines. Anti-inflammatory cytokines (e.g., IL-1ra and IL-10) may be released.

Taken together, this indicates that immune surveillance is enhanced. There is an enhanced potential for immune cells to come into contact with a pathogen, respond, and get rid of it.

During Heavy Exertion:

Cortisol, which is known to suppress the immune system, is elevated. TNF-α and IL-6, inflammatory cytokines released from the muscle, are significantly elevated.

Function of neutrophils in nasal passages is suppressed for up to a week following intense, long-duration physical activity.

Certain antibodies (IgA) from nasal passages are suppressed for up to 18 hours after intense exercise.

Conclusion:

The acute effect of short-term exercise (5 to 60 minutes) causes very few **functional** changes in the immune system (total circulating number of cells may increase significantly). However, exercising for 60 minutes or greater, especially at high intensities (70 to 80% Vo_2max or greater) alters the immune system for 3 to 72 hours post exercise.

The "Open Window" Hypothesis

During moderate as well as severe exercise, the immune system is enhanced, but severe exercise is followed by immunodepression.

This immunodepression which may last for 1 to 24 hours makes the individual more susceptible to infection.

Review Questions: Chapter 13: Part One

(For true and false questions that are false, indicate what would make the question true)

1. What gland is considered a neuroendocrine gland?

    a. Testes

    b. Pineal Gland

    c. Hypothalamus

    d. Pituitary Gland

    e. Adrenal Gland

2. Exocrine glands contain secretory ducts that carry substances directly to the target tissue or compartment. An example of an exocrine gland would be:

    a. upper GI glands

    b. sweat glands

    c. anterior and posterior pituitary gland

    d. a and b

    e. all of the above

3. True or False:

    A steroid derived hormone has its receptor located on the cell membrane of the target tissue.

4. In response to high hormone levels, cell receptors will **up-regulate/ down-regulate.** This **maximizes/minimizes** the effect of the hormone on the target cell.

5. True or False:

    All protein hormones are released in a pulsatile manner.

6. The _____ secretes many hormones including FSH, LH, GH, prolactin, and ACTH.

7. In response to growth hormone stimulation, the _____ synthesizes _____.

    a. anterior pituitary gland; IGF I and IGF II

    b. posterior pituitary gland; IGF I and IGF II

    c. liver; IGF I and IGF II

    d. hypothalamus; testosterone

8. Hormone release by _____ stimulation occurs when levels of ions and nutrients change in the blood, bile, or other body fluid.

    a. hormonal

    b. humoral

    c. neural

Chapter 13—Exercise and the Endocrine System   261

d. a and b

e. b and c

f. a, b, and c

9. ACTH release from the anterior pituitary acts on the adrenal cortex to release glucocorticoids. This is an example of _____ stimulation.

a. hormonal

b. humoral

c. neural

d. a and b

e. b and c

f. a, b, and c.

10. What does the adrenal medulla secrete in response to preganglionic sympathetic nervous system fibers?

11. What is the definition of a tropic hormone?

12. True or False:

Prolactin is a tropic hormone.

13. Which of the anterior pituitary hormones are tropic?

14. What is another name for GHIH (Growth Hormone Inhibiting Hormone)? Where is it produced and what structure does it affect?

15. True or False:

Growth Hormone has anti-insulin effects such as increased fatty acid mobilization and decreased uptake of glucose (to maintain blood glucose levels).

16. The **anterior/posterior** pituitary gland is anatomically connected to the hypothalamus.

17. What two hormones are released from the posterior pituitary gland? What are their primary functions?

18. The catecholamines are released from the _____, while glucocorticoids, mineralocorticoids, and androgens are released from the _____.

a. adrenal cortex, adrenal medulla

b. adrenal medulla, adrenal cortex

c. adrenal cortex, adrenal cortex

d. adrenal medulla, adrenal medulla

e. none of these

19. True or False:

Generally, as exercise intensity increases, catecholamine levels increase.

262   Chapter 13—Exercise and the Endocrine System

20. _____ is the precursor of _____.

   a. epinephrine, norepinephrine

   b. norepinephrine, epinephrine

21. Aldosterone causes increased **potassium/sodium** reabsorption in the kidney, resulting in **increased/decreased/no effect** blood volume, **increased/decreased/no effect on** blood pressure, and **increased/decreased/no effect on** cardiac output.

22. A decrease in sodium and increase in potassium in the blood will cause what hormone to be released?

23. True or False:

   DHEA (dehydroepiandrosterone) has similar effects as testosterone.

24. The female triad consists of what three co-existing medical conditions?

25. In what four ways does estrogen have a protective effect on bone?

26. The release of insulin from the _____ causes an _____ in blood glucose, and the release of glucagon from the _____ causes a _____ in blood glucose. Thus, insulin and glucagon have opposing functions.

27. True or False:

   Anti Diuretic Hormone would be expected to decrease during exercise in hot environments.

28. List the diagnostic criteria for Diabetes Mellitus.

29. True or False:

   A type one diabetic is exercising in the human performance laboratory and is experiencing symptoms of hypoglycemia. This is due to the insufficient production of insulin.

30. How does exercise function to reduce the risk of developing Type 2 diabetes? What is/are the mechanism(s) involved?

31. What is the primary concern for a person with Type 1 Diabetes when exercising?

32. What are several benefits of lifelong exercise for patients with Type 2 Diabetes?

33. Moderate exercise training has been shown to **increase/decrease** oneís chance of developing an upper respiratory tract infection while strenuous exercise training has been shown to **increase/decrease** the same.

34. Define the open window hypothesis.

35. What supplement has been shown to attenuate the negative effects of exercise on the immune system? What is the proposed theory for why this happens?

Chapter 13—Exercise and the Endocrine System   263

Exercise and Immune Review Questions

1. Briefly discuss the differences between the innate and acquired immune systems.

2. a. Give three examples of the innate immune system:

    b. Give three examples of the acquired immune system:

3. The _____ cells are often called the "quarter back" of immune regulation because they respond to antigen presenting cells causing many other immune cells to become active.

    a. T cells

    b. B cells

    c. Macrophages

    d. NK cells

    e. Plasma cells

4. a. _____ is one of the most striking and consistent changes observed during exercise.

    b. Define this term:

5. Briefly discuss what happens to circulating lymphocyte numbers immediately following high intensity exercise.

264   Chapter 13—Exercise and the Endocrine System

6. Give one possible cause for your answer in number 5.

7. Salivary levels of _____ have been shown to be lower following high intensity exercise.

    a. IgM

    b. IgA

    c. IgG

    d. B cells

    e. T cells

8. Briefly define the J-shaped relationship between upper respiratory tract infections and exercise intensity.

9. Define the Open Window Hypothesis:

Chapter 13

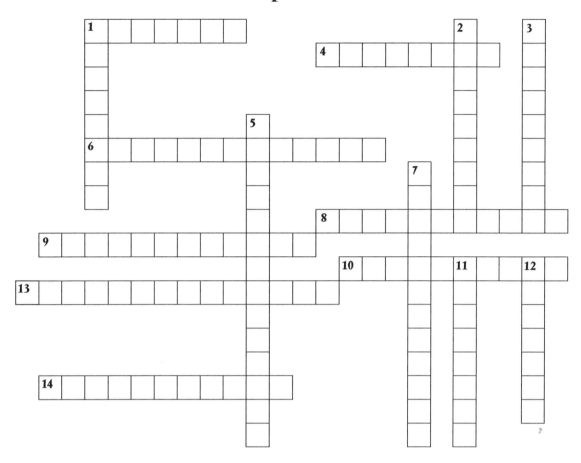

ACROSS

1. Hormone that assists in digestion and absorption of nutrients.
4. Type of gland that contains secretory ducts.
6. Also called somatotropin, represents a family of polypeptides that promote cell division and proliferation throughout the body.
8. Represents almost 95% of all mineralocorticoids produced.
9. The state whereby target cells form more receptors in response to increasing hormone levels.
10. Another name for the pituitary gland.
13. A glycoprotein that stimulates the bone marrow's production of red blood cells.
14. Hormone that promotes aldosterone secretion and increases blood pressure.

DOWN

1. Hormone that raises blood glucose levels.
2. Type of gland that posses no ducts.
3. Hormone that initiates and supports milk secretion from the mammary glands.
5. Principle neurotransmitter released from the sympathetic nervous system.
7. The most important androgen secreted by the interstitial cells of the testes.
11. Chemical substances synthesized by specific host glands that enter the bloodstream for transport throughout the body.
12. Hormone that lowers blood glucose levels.

Unit 2

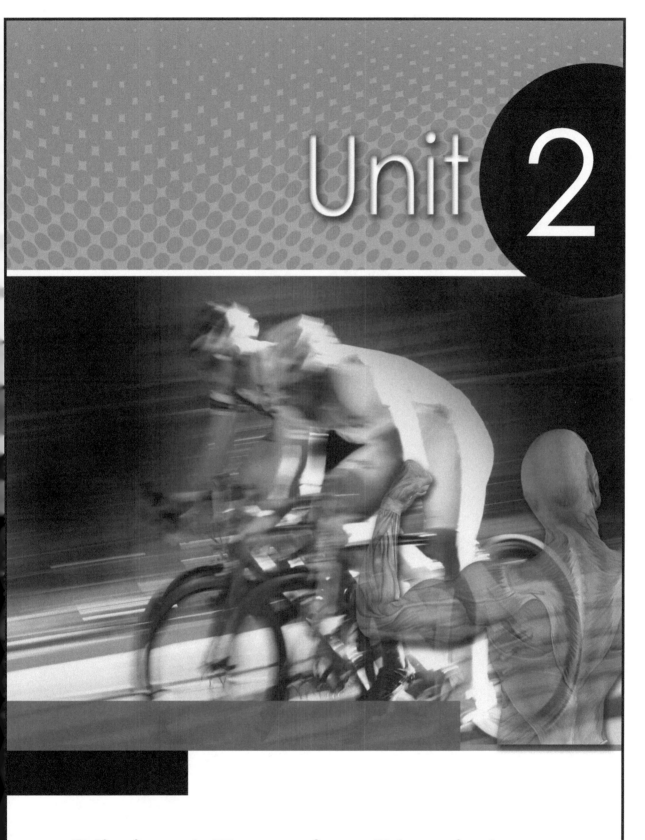

Clinical Exercise Physiology

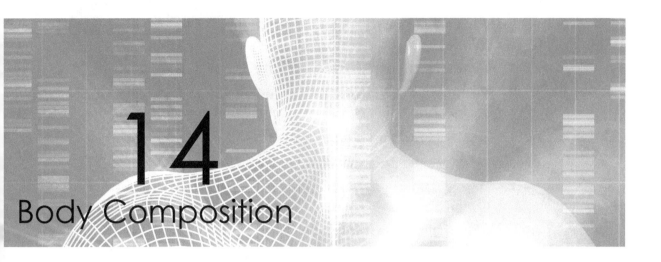

14
Body Composition

METHODS TO DETERMINE "OVERWEIGHTNESS"

Height-Weight tables relate average stature with lowest mortality

- Use unvalidated estimates of body frame
- DO not consider specific cause of death
- Specific focus on mortality, DO not consider morbidity (quality of health)
- Developed from data derived from primarily in Caucasian populations
- Unvalidated and do not consider body composition

BODY MASS INDEX (BMI)

BMI = weight (kg) / height (m²)

BMI greater or equal to 25 is overweight and BMI greater or equal to 30 is obese.

Curve–linear relationship with all-cause mortality

- Higher, but moderate associations with body fat and disease risk
- Not validated for children
- Assumes BMI remains independent of age, gender, race
- No indication of fat patterning
- Factors other than excess body fat, such as bone, muscle mass, and increased plasma volume induced by exercise training affect the numerator of the BMI equation.

◄ Can the BMI be too low? How could this affect health especially in women?

COMPOSITION OF THE HUMAN BODY

Essential and Storage Fat

Essential fat—consists of fat in the heart, lungs, spleen, kidneys, intestines, muscles, and lipid-rich tissues of the central nervous system.

- Required for normal function
- Includes sex specific fat in females

Storage fat—includes fat primarily in adipose tissue. (visceral and subcutaneous deposits)

- Similar proportional distribution in men and women (12%, 15%)

Reference man: 12% storage fat and 3% essential fat

Reference woman: 15% storage fat and 12% essential fat

FAT-FREE MASS AND LEAN BODY MASS

Lean Body Mass (LBM)—includes non–sex-specific essential fat equivalent to approximately 3% of body mass

- Fat-free mass (FFM)—body mass devoid of all extractable fat
  - Bone, muscle, connective tissue

MINIMAL LEANNESS STANDARDS

A biologically lower limit beyond which a person's body cannot decrease with out impairing health status or altering normal physiological functions.

Reference Man & Woman

Is a useful statistical comparison from which thousands of individuals were measured.

Partitions body mass into LBM: muscle, bone, essential fat, body fat: storage essential

- Reference man is taller, weighs more, has a heavier skeleton, and lower body fat.
- Predominantly due to hormonal differences

Average Body Fat:

- Young adult men: 12 to 15%
- Young adult women: 25 to 28%
- "No systematic evaluation exists for body composition of the general population to warrant establishing norms or precise recommended values for body composition"
- The general trend indicates a tendency for percentage body fat to steadily increase with advancing age

Computing Fat Mass:

- Fat mass = body mass × (% fat/100)
- Fat-free body mass = body mass − fat mass

Determining Goal Body Weight:

Goal body weight (kg) = fat-free body mass / (1.00 − desired %fat)

ASSESSING OF BODY COMPOSITION

Direct assessment to evaluate body composition

Cadaver analysis—dissection

Indirect assessment to evaluate body composition:

- Hydrostatic weighing using Archimedes' principle
- Skinfold thickness and girth measurements
- X-ray and magnetic resonance imaging
- Total body electrical conductivity or bioimpedance
- Near-infrared interactance
- Ultrasound
- Computed tomography
- Air plethysmography

Densitometry

1. Hydrostatic (underwater) weighing is based on Archimedes' principle

    - Measuring mass per unit volume
    - Weight of body on land, weight of body in water, density of water
    - A person's weight in water is a function of the individual's body density

    Muscle > density than water (1.1 g/cm^3 vs. 1.0 g/cm^3)

    Fat < density than water (0.9 g/cm^3).

    Body density = dry weight / [((dry weight − wet weight) / water density) − RV − 0.1]

    Whole-body density estimates body fat percentage:

    Siri equation:

    $$\text{Percentage body fat} = (495 \, / \, \text{body density}) - 450$$

Chapter 14—Body Composition   273

Assumes:

Two-component model of body composition

Each of these densities remains relatively constant among individuals

Densities of the lean tissue components of bone and muscle remained the same among individuals

Limitations to estimating body fat

Formulas assume the density of FFM remain a constant across the population

- represent averages for young and middle-aged adults

- vary among individuals and groups

Average density is higher in African Americans and Hispanics overestimating FFM underestimating body fat.

Changes in mineral density in young children and the elderly

Modification of the Siri equation computes percentage body fat from body density for blacks:

Percentage body fat = (437.4 / body density) − 392.8

2. Bod Pod

A procedure based on air displacement

Subjects enter a sealed chamber that determines body volume by measuring the initial volume of the empty chamber and then the volume with the person inside

- Vol = Vi−Vs

- Takes into account lung volume

Body volume is combined with body weight (mass) in order to determine body density.

The technique then estimates the percentage of body fat and LBM through known equations (for the density of fat and FFM).

Anthropometry

1. Skinfold

Approximately 50% of body fat is stored beneath the skin (subcutaneous)

Measure subcutaneous fat at various sites and determine percent body fat with various equations.

Sites include:

- Triceps: Vertical fold at posterior midline of right upper arm, halfway between tip of shoulder and tip of elbow

- Subscapular: Oblique fold, below right scapula's lower tip

- Iliac: Slightly oblique fold, just above the right hipbone (crest of ileum); the fold follows the natural diagonal line

- Abdominal: Vertical fold 1 inch to the right of umbilicus

- Thigh: Vertical fold at the midline of right thigh, two-third the distance from the middle of the patella to the hip

- Chest: Diagonal fold on the anterior axillary line

- Biceps: Vertical fold at right upper arm's midline

Advantages:

- The procedure has some degree of repeatability.

- It gives meaningful information about body fat distribution and relative changes that may occur following an intervention.

Skinfold Precautions:

Skinfold test should not be measured immediately after exercise. Exercise increases extracellular water accumulation in subcutaneous tissue resulting in increased skin fold thickness.

For extremely obese people, a skinfold test is not likely to be possible due to the inability to apply the calipers and is not recommended for this population.

Equations used to predict total body fat from subcutaneous skinfold measurement are based on adult cadaver studies of small sample size and may not be accurate for all populations (elderly, children, race, etc.)

2. Girth Measurement

- Right upper arm (biceps): arm straight and extended in front of the body; measurement taken at midpoint between the shoulder and the elbow

- Right forearm: maximum girth with arm extended in front of the body

- Abdomen: 1 inch above the umbilicus

- Buttocks: maximum protrusion with heels together

- Right thigh: upper thigh, just below the buttocks

- Right calf: widest girth midway between ankle and knee

Bioelectrical Impedance Analysis (BIA)

Principle—electronic pulses that passes through muscle and fat at different rates.

- Passes rapidly through hydrated FFM and EC water

  - lower electrical resistance due to greater electrolyte content

- Passes slowly through fat or bone tissues

  - higher electrical resistance

Impedance to electric current flow is calculated:

Chapter 14—Body Composition   275

In practice, a small constant current, typically 400 uA at a fixed frequency, usually 50 kHz, is passed between electrodes spanning the body, and the voltage drop between electrodes provides a measure of impedance.

- Represents a noninvasive, safe, relatively easy, and reliable means to assess total body water
- Requires standardized conditions: electrode placement, body position, hydration status, plasma osmolality and sodium concentration, skin temperature, recent physical activity, and previous food and beverage intake

Problems:

- Hydration effects electrolytes and thus current flow
  - Decreased hydration = decreased body fat
- Less accurate than skinfolds/girths
  - Lacks sensitivity to detect small body comp changes
- Poor for athletic populations
  - Need sport specific equations

Near Infrared Interactance

Principles of light absorption and reflection

Fiber optic probe emits low-energy infrared light

Shifts in wavelength computed into FFM and %BF

Ultrasound

Electrical energy from a probe is emitted as high-frequency sound waves

Reflect fat–muscle interface to produce and ECHO which is imaged on the screen

High reliability

Total or segmental subcutaneous AT and FFM

Particularly useful with obese individuals

Computed Tomography (CT)

Detailed cross-sectional 2D radiographic image

X-ray beam passing through tissues of different densities

Pictorial and quantitative data:

Total tissue area

Total fat and muscle area

Thickness and volume of tissues

MRI

Noninvasive assessment of body's tissue compartments

Electromagnetic radiation excites hydrogen nuclei in water and lipid

Signal is transformed into visual representations

Quantifies total and subcutaneous adipose tissue

Can indicate changes in muscle mass

Dual X-Ray Absorptiometry

Accurately quantifies fat and non-bone regional LBM, including the mineral content of the body's deeper bony structures.

Two low-energy x-ray beams penetrate to a depth of approximately 30 cm

Reconstructs attenuated x-ray beams to produce an image of underlying tissues

- Quantify bone mineral content, total fat mass, and FFM

Excellent agreement with hydrostatic weighing and skinfolds

Review Questions for Chapter 14

(For true and false questions that are false, indicate what would make the question true)

1. Mathematically define BMI.

2. A person is classified as being overweight with a BMI ≥ _____, and classified as obese with a BMI ≥ _____.

3. True or False:

   Having an extremely low BMI (i.e., ≤18 for women) is healthy and reduces the risk of all cause mortality.

4. True or False:

   A BMI of greater than 25 means an individual has excessive abdominal fat.

5. Define storage fat and give the values for the reference man and women.

6. Define essential fat and give the values for the reference man and woman.

7. List the five levels of the five-level model of body composition.

8. Briefly, describe the principle behind hydrostatic weighing.

Chapter 14—Body Composition   279

9. The specific purpose of hydrostatic weighing is to determine _____.

    a. Body weight

    b. Body volume

    c. Body fat

    d. Body water

    e. None of these

10. True or False:

The rationale for using skinfolds to estimate body fat comes from the fact that 75% of all body fat is subcutaneous.

11. True or False:

Similar formulas are used for children and adults to determine body fat from skinfold measurements.

12. True or False:

The Bod Pod is an example of densitometry.

13. Briefly, describe the purpose of bioelectrical impedance and how this procedure may be used for estimating body composition.

14. True or False:

Dehydration will result in an inaccurate BIA reading and will give an artificially high measure of body fat.

15. Why is it important to measure waist/hip ratios? What can this tell you about the individual's health?

280   Chapter 14—Body Composition

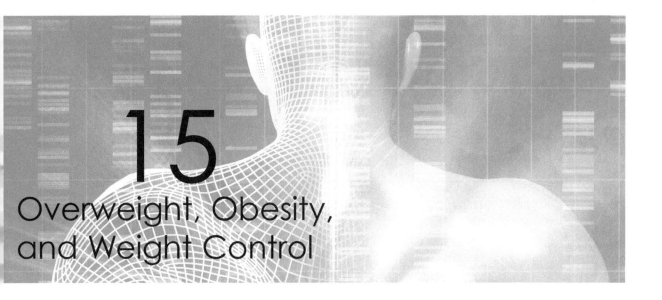

15
Overweight, Obesity, and Weight Control

The number of individuals who are considered overweight or obese is on the rise in the United States and worldwide and increasing at an alarming rate.

Obesity—both morbid and not—has been linked to a number of serious diseases.

OVERWEIGHT AND OBESITY: BY THE NUMBERS:

In last two decades, prevalence increased by 50 to 100% among adults, and three-fold among children and adolescents

62% of the U.S. populations are overweight, of these, 30% are obese

Higher in specific subgroups

- i.e., African American women have an 80% and 50% prevalence of overweight and obesity, respectively

29% of the U.S. adults report no regular physical activity

70% of American adults struggle to lose weight

$40 billion/year industry

Enough food is produced in the United States to supply 3,800 calories every day to each man, woman, and child in the country.

- Daily recommended for average adult 2000 to 2500 calories

Between 1970 and 2000, the typical American man increased his caloric intake by 168 calories a day while the average woman added 335 calories a day.

There are numerous health risks associated with being overweight.

There is no unanimity for the terminology describing overweight, overfat, and obesity

- "Obesity means having too much body fat."

- "Overweight means weighing too much."

BMI Definitions:

Overweight (25 to 29.9)

Obesity (=> 30)

How does body composition assessment play into these definitions?

In most medical literature:

Overweight describes an overly fat condition (BMI $\geq$ 25)

Obese refers to individuals at the extreme of the overweight continuum. (BMI $\geq$ 30)

A. Class one: BMI: 30–34.9

B. Class two: BMI: 35–39.9

C. Class three: BMI $\geq$ 40

Obesity is a process that does not occur over night but usually takes many years. (Energy intake **chronically** exceeds energy expenditure.)

Mindless Eating:

- Dr. Brian Wansick is an American professor in the fields of consumer behavior and nutritional science

- Currently the Director of the Cornell Food and Brand Lab

Do individuals gain or lose weight quickly? Why?

- Homeostatic mechanisms keep this difference very close to zero.

- For example, nonobese adults ingest about 900,000 kcal of food per year

- Approximately 3,500 kcal of chemical energy is stored in 1 lb of adipose tissue.

- If intake exceeded expenditure by 2% daily for 1 year, the result would be an increase of 18,000 kcal or approximately 5 lb.

What causes obesity?

"American society has become 'obesogenic,' characterized by environment that promote increased food intake, nonhealthy foods, and physical inactivity

Main problem is an imbalance in energy balance equation (Energy intake = Energy expenditure = Energy balance).

Simple rule of thumb—To lose 1 lb of fat, must decrease intake of energy by 3,500 kcal or increase expenditure of energy by 3,500 kcal or a combination of both.

However, treatment directed toward long-term reduction of body weight is largely ineffective, and 90 to 95% of persons who lose weight subsequently regain it.

The expenditure side of the equation consists of:

Energy expended during rest (basal metabolism rate or BMR)

Energy used to break down food (thermogenesis)

Energy used during physical activity

When a person consumes more calories than the energy they use, the body stores the extra calories in fat cells.

OBESITY: COMPLEX INTERACTION OF MANY FACTORS

Being overweight and obese is the result of an interaction of genetic, environmental, metabolic, physiologic, behavior, social, and possibly even racial influences.

a. Genetics influences:

Difficult to quantify role of genetics and environment

Recent studies of thousands of preteen twins found that genetic factors have a considerable influence on BMI and obesity.

Estimates for the role of genetics on BMI have been reported to be as low as 25% to as high as 90%.

However, a recent large family study has put the heritability estimate at approximately 67%.

A heritability estimate of this magnitude indicates that the genetic component for body weight is not that much below that for body height.

Do your genes influence weight gain through overfeeding? Weight lose through dieting? Weight loss through exercise?

Genetics also determines the number of fat cells a person has.

Mutant gene?

Leptin theory—leptin levels rise as the cells store more fat. This increase in leptin levels decreases appetite. Low levels of leptin make you feel hungry.

Chapter 15—Overweight, Obesity, and Weight Control   283

However, most obese people do not have any abnormalities in the coding sequences for leptin, and in fact, plasma leptin concentrations are **increased** in obese humans in direct proportion to body fat.

- Human obesity therefore resembles a condition of **leptin resistance.**

- Some studies have indicated that leptin resistance may precede insulin resistance.

- Several agonists cause release from the adipocyte:

  - TNF-α, other pro-inflammatory cytokines, insulin, glucose, and estrogens

- Involved in processes such as growth, metabolic control, immune regulation, insulin sensitivity, and reproduction

- Leptin has recently been demonstrated to have profound effects on skeletal muscle fatty acid (FA) metabolism resulting in an increase in the capacity to oxidize FA and lower intramuscular stores and improve insulin sensitivity.

- It has been hypothesized that one of the major roles of leptin is to **prevent lipid overload,** or **lipid toxicity**, in peripheral tissues.

- Recent evidence points to the development of **leptin resistance** in skeletal muscle associated with obesity. This can lead to the redistribution of FA transporters to the membrane resulting in enhanced FA uptake in excess of that which can be oxidized, and lipid deposition (leptin resistance may precede insulin resistance).

Adipocytokines

- Recent studies have shown that fat tissue is not a simple energy storage organ, but exerts important **endocrine** and **immune** functions.

- Obesity is characterized by increased plasma C-reactive proteins levels as well as dysregulated cytokine production by monocytes, lymphocytes, and other immune cells (**state of general inflammation**).

- Obesity is also associated with the presence of *endothelial and vascular dysfunction*.

- Adipocytokines: bioactive mediator factors released by adipocytes or cells within the adipose tissue, some of which have been linked to atherosclerosis and cardiovascular morbidity.

- The effects of adipocytokines on vascular function, immune regulation, and adipocyte metabolism make them key players in the pathogenesis of metabolic syndrome.

METABOLIC SYNDROME

- *Metabolic syndrome* is a cluster of conditions that occur together increasing the risk of heart disease, stroke, and diabetes.

- Approximately **47 million** adults in the United States have metabolic syndrome.

- Over **300 million** people world wide.

- Three or more of the following criteria:
  - Central obesity (waist circumference >102 cm in men; >88 cm in women)
  - Hypertriglyceridemia ($\geq$1.69 mmol/L)
  - Low HDL (<1.04 mmol/L in men; <1.29 mmol/L in women)
  - Hypertension ($\geq$130/85 mmHg)
  - High fasting blood glucose ($\geq$6.1 mmol/L)
- Potential clinical outcome:
  - CVD
  - Type 2 diabetes
  - Polycystic ovary syndrome
  - Fatty liver
  - Cholesterol gallstones
  - Asthma
  - Sleep disturbances
  - Certain cancers

Adiponectin

- Is a 247 amino acid protein (30-kDa).
- Considered to be a "beneficial" cytokine. (anti-inflammatory, vasculo-protective, anti-diabetic effects).
- Levels in individuals with insulin resistance and diabetes have been shown to be reduced.
- Administration has been shown to cause glucose lowering and reduced insulin resistance.
- Certain inflammatory mediators (e.g., TNFα, IL-6) have been shown to decrease levels.
- Is lowered in the obese individual even though it comes primarily from adipose tissue.
- A population-based study showed an inverse relationship between adiponectin and small LDL densities.
- Appears to inhibit the NFkB pathway (important in the induction of cytokines including TNF-α) and therefore lowers inflammation by lowering inflammatory cytokine production.
- In contrast to leptin, adiponectin has consistently been shown to have protective vascular effects.

Uncoupling Proteins

May play a role in the regulation of energy metabolism by uncoupling respiration from phosphorylation leading to the generation of heat instead of ATP.

A certain polymorphism (BcII) in this gene has been significantly associated with increases in the percentage of body fat.

Chapter 15—Overweight, Obesity, and Weight Control   285

Beta Adrenergic Receptors

Human beta-2 adrenergic receptor gene:

- Encodes a 413-amino acid protein which controls glycogen breakdown and lipid metabolism.

- Under normal conditions, it is the dominating lipolytic adrenergic receptor subtype.

- It is down regulated in the subcutaneous adipose tissue of obese subjects.

Abnormality in this gene is associated with:

- a reduced metabolic rate

- increased body weight

- increased subcutaneous fat

- decreased weight loss following programs of diet and exercise

b. Influence of racial factors

Differences in food and exercise habits, cultural attitudes toward weight may explain some of the differences between specific races.

Differences in resting energy expenditure (REE).

- African-American women 10% lower REE, 19% lower physical activity energy expenditure, and greater prevalence of obesity than Caucasian women.

Is the main influence race or the environment?

c. Physical inactivity

Studies have clearly shown that regular recreational or occupational physical activity reduces weight and prevents weight gain following weight-loss interventions.

Can you have cardiovascular fitness but still be overweight?

- A study in men found that all-cause mortality was lower in individuals who were physically fit but had excessive body fat compared with those unfit but of normal weight.

Sedentary habits have contributed significantly to the overweight and obesity epidemic.

286   Chapter 15—Overweight, Obesity, and Weight Control

DETERMINING OVERFATNESS:

Must consider:

1. Percentage of body fat
2. Distribution of body fat
3. Size and number of individual adipocytes

1. Criteria for excessive body fat:

2. Regional fat distribution:

- The distribution of body fat is an independent risk factor (independent of total body fat) in children, adolescents, and adults.
- Most males present with central or android-type obesity
- Most females present with peripheral or gynoid-type obesity

Central obesity is a risk factor for the metabolic syndrome (Syndrome X) and increases the chances of developing:

- Hyperinsulinemia (insulin resistance)
- Glucose intolerance
- Type 2 diabetes
- Endometrial cancer
- Hypertriglyceridemia
- Negatively altered lipoprotein profile
- Hypertension
- Atherosclerosis

Lipoprotein lipase (LPL) affects body fat distribution

- Lipoprotein lipase is a rate-limiting enzyme that facilitates uptake and storage by fat cells (adipocytes)
- LPL plays a role in gender differences in fat patterning.

  Females have greater LPL activity in hips, thighs, and breasts.

  Males have higher LPL activity in abdomen.

3. Adipocyte size and number

Adipose tissue mass can increase in one of two ways:

a. Hypertrophy
b. Hyperplasia

Chapter 15—Overweight, Obesity, and Weight Control   287

There is a major difference in the number of adipocytes between severely obese and non-obese individuals.

Effects of weight loss:

- Adipocyte **size** decreases, while **number** remains the same

Effects of weight gain:

- Moderate weight gain results from increased adipocyte size.
- Severe weight gain may be accompanied by an increase in adipocyte number.

Approximately 10% of fat cells are renewed annually. Neither adipocyte death nor generation rate is altered in early onset obesity, suggesting a tight regulation of fat cell number in this condition during adulthood.

Important times for adipocyte development:

- Cell size and number increase with development
- Between ages 1 and 6, cell size triples

What are the important times during development when fat cells increase in number?

Two general types of obesity:

1. *Childhood onset*

   Adipose tissue contains four or five times the number (hyperplasia) of cells as normal.

   Have an increase in the number of fat cells in the last three months of fetal development, the first year of life, and during adolescent growth spurt.

   Estimated that 80% of obese children remain obese.

   Severe obesity is associated with hyperplasia of fat cells.

   In formula-fed infants, weight gain during the first week of life may be a critical determinant for the development of obesity several decades later.

2. *Adult onset*:

   Usually caused by an increase in fat cell size (hypertrophy).

   However, there is an upper limit to the size a fat cell can become.

   If exceed this limit you can increase the number (severe obesity).

   Adipose cell believed to be responsible for mild to moderate obesity in adulthood.

ENERGY BALANCE: INPUT VERSUS OUTPUT

The first law of thermodynamics, in essences, states that body weight will remain stable if energy intake equals energy expenditure.

Dieting for weight control

Long-term success depends on the degree of obesity at the start of intervention.

The potential for successful long-term weight loss maintenance generally varies inversely with the initial degree of fatness.

Weight Loss Plans:

Goal should be to lose 1 to 2 lb per week.

(1 lb of body fat = about 3,500 calories)

New recommendations are for obese individuals to reduce initial body weight by 5 to 15%.

Avoid crash starvation diets.

Best long-term weight loss is accomplished by combining exercise with a diet consisting of 0.9 g of protein/kg body weight, 60% complex carbohydrates, and <30% fat (at least 50% unsaturated).

Most important consideration is to reduce total calories.

Have a support group.

How does weight lose through caloric restriction affect lean body mass?

Successful Weight Management

Studies show that people who lost atleast 10% of their body weight and kept the weight off for more than 1 year share several characteristics, including:

- Exercising for at least 1 hour each day
- Eating a low-fat, low-calorie diet
- Eating breakfast each day
- Weighing themselves regularly and often
- Eating the same diet on weekends as they do on weekdays

National Weight Control Registry:

- Is the largest database of individuals (784) who successfully achieved prolonged weight loss
- Average weight loss of individuals equaled 66 lbs (minimum requirement of 30 lbs) for average of 5.5 years
- Approximately 50% had one obese parent/approximately 25% had two
- All used behavioral approaches to food intake
- All maintained at least 30-lb weight loss for 1 year
- Regarding weight-loss methods, 89% reported **modifying food intake** and maintained relatively **high levels of physical activity** (2,800 kcal weekly on average)

Long-Term Success

It is important to tell patients that weight loss improves disease risk biomarkers (modest weight loss = health benefit).

What is the Set-point theory and does it affect weight loss?

- The ability to lose weight is partially under the control of the hypothalamus
- Resting metabolism decreases with weight loss
- Biologic feedback mechanism may exist between the brain and body's fat stores
- Exercise may lower ones set-point!

Dieting Extremes:

Low carbohydrate–ketogenic diets:

i.e., Atkins diet:

Cut all CHO and eat all the fat they want.

Avoid foods such as beans, breads, most fruits, starchy vegetables, and foods with whole grain.

The thought is that by removing CHO, the body will enter a state of ketosis (burning of fats and food cravings disappear).

Very difficult diet to maintain, often causes fatigue, short-term weight loss as a result of dehydration.

High-protein diets:

Very-low calorie diets (VLCD)

Factors that affect weight loss:

- Early weight loss is largely water (up to 70% in the first week).

- Dieters lose the quantity of body fat regardless of fluid intake (should not restrict water intake)

- Longer term caloric deficit promotes fat loss.

Exercise:

Is the most variable side of energy expenditure equation (5 to 40% of daily energy expenditure).

May help to regulate appetite and lower fat weight.

The primary goal in weight loss is the total work accomplished, therefore, low-intensity, long-duration exercise is as good as high-intensity, short-duration exercise in expending calories.

The existent literature appears to provide little evidence that exercise **alone** is a **potent strategy** for weight loss.

A review of several studies showed that exercise **alone** showed a 1.15 kg weight loss in a typical 12-week program.

ACSM Position Stand on *"Appropriate intervention strategies for weight loss and prevention of weight regain for adults,"* acknowledges that there is little evidence to suggest exercise **alone** will provide the amount of weight loss similar to that generally achieved by diet restriction.

Exercise **may** not cause increase in food intake to balance additional energy expenditure although the evidence on this is mixed.

The discrepancy between the energy expenditure of exercise for men and women may contribute to the observation that women generally lose less weight than men in response to exercise.

In addition, it appears that women involved in exercise training programs **may** compensate by increasing caloric intake more so then men.

CDC 2008 PHYSICAL ACTIVITY GUIDELINES FOR AMERICANS

150 minutes of **moderate-intensity aerobic activity** (i.e., brisk walking) every week

And

Muscle-strengthening activities on two or more days a week that work all muscle groups (legs, hips, back, abdomen, chest, shoulders, and arms)

Or

75 minutes of **vigorous-intensity aerobic activities** (i.e., jogging or running) every week

And

Muscle-strengthening activities on two or more days a week

Or

An equivalent mix of ***moderate and vigorous-intensity aerobic activity***

And

Muscle-strengthening activities on two or more days a week

For Even *Greater* Health Benefits including Weight Loss

300 minutes of ***moderate-intensity aerobic activity*** (i.e., brisk walking) every week

And

Muscle-strengthening activities on two or more days a week that work all muscle groups (legs, hips, back, abdomen, chest, shoulders, and arms)

Or

150 minutes of ***vigorous-intensity aerobic activities*** (i.e., jogging or running) every week

And

Muscle-strengthening activities on two or more days a week

Or

An equivalent mix of ***moderate- and vigorous-intensity aerobic activity***

And

Muscle-strengthening activities on two or more days a week

10 minutes at a time is fine

150 minutes each week sounds like a lot of time, but an individual does not have to do it all at once. Not only is it best to **spread the activity out during the week**, but it can be broken **into smaller chunks of time during the day**. As long as the person is doing the activity at a moderate or vigorous effort for **at least 10 minutes at a time.**

CDC 2008 PHYSICAL ACTIVITY GUIDELINES FOR AMERICANS (CHILDREN)

Children and adolescents should do 60 minutes (1 hour) or more of physical activity each day.

Aerobic activity should make up most of a child's 60 or more minutes of physical activity each day.

Include ***muscle-strengthening activities***, such as gymnastics or push ups, at least three days per week as part of a child's 60 or more minutes

Include ***bone-strengthening activities***, such as jumping rope or running, at least three days per week as part of a child's 60 or more minutes.

DIET PLUS EXERCISE: THE IDEAL COMBINATION

What is spot reduction and does it work?

Possible gender difference

- Men appear to respond better to weight loss interventions.
- May be due to fat patterning

WEIGHT LOSS RECOMMENDATIONS FOR WRESTLERS AND OTHER POWER ATHLETES

- The recommendation is 5% body fat as a lower limit (7% for those under 16)

Gaining weight: the competitive athlete's dilemma

BEHAVIORAL THEORIES AND STRATEGIES FOR PROMOTING PHYSICAL ACTIVITY CHANGE

Understanding Each Persons Why

- In the past, prescribing physical activity and exercise typically consisted of explaining the many wonderful benefits of physical activity and the harmful health consequences of being physically inactive.
- Very little attention given to the individuals willingness and desire to adopt and or change their behavior.
- It is now routine practice to identify the persons perceptions, attitudes and beliefs about physical activity when performing their initial assessment.
- Numerous demographic factors (e.g., age, gender, socioeconomic status, education, ethnicity) are consistently related to the likelihood that an individual will exercise on a regular basis.
- These factors suggest who might benefit most from the exercise intervention.

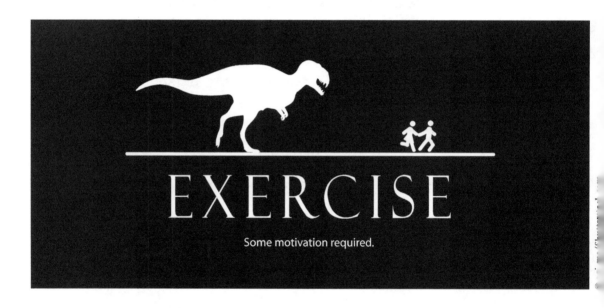

THEORETICAL FOUNDATIONS FOR UNDERSTANDING EXERCISE BEHAVIOR

- Social Cognitive Theory
- Transtheoretical Model
- Health Belief Model
- Self-determination Theory
- Theory of Planned Behavior
- Social Ecological Models

SOCIAL COGNITIVE THEORY (SCT) AND SELF-EFFICACY

- Central to SCT is the concept of ***self-efficacy***, which refers to one's beliefs in her or his capability to successfully complete a course of action such as exercise.

- ***Task self-efficacy*** refers to an individual's belief that she or he can actually do the behavior in question, whereas ***barriers self-efficacy*** refers to whether an individual believes she or he can regularly exercise in the face of common barriers such as lack of time, poor weather, and feeling tired.

- The higher the sense of efficacy, the greater the effort, persistence, and resilience an individual will exhibit, especially when faced with barriers or challenges.

- Self efficacy is one of the most consistently found correlates of physical activity in adults and youth.

- ***Outcome expectations and expectancies*** are key concepts of SCT. Anticipatory results of a behavior and the value one puts on these results.

- If specific outcomes are valued, then behavior change is more likely to occur.

- For example, if an overweight adults who wants to lose weight and believes that walking will help is more likely to start and maintain a walking program.

- What is the most common reason people report for starting an exercise program? Is this good or bad in terms of exercise adherence?

Self-regulation or self-control is another important concept in SCT. This refers to a person's ability to:

- Set goals

- Monitor progress toward those goals

- Problem solve when faced with barriers

- Engage in self-reward

Transtheoretical Model

- The Transtheoretical Model (TTM) was developed as a framework for understanding behavior change and is one of the most popular methods for promoting exercise behavior.

- Individuals are at different stages of readiness to make behavioral changes and thus require tailored interventions.

The stages of change

- Precontemplation

- Contemplation

- Preparation

- Action

- Maintenance

HEALTH BELIEF MODEL

- Theorizes that one's beliefs about whether they are susceptible to disease and their perceptions of the benefits of trying to avoid it influence their readiness to act

- The theory is grounded in the notion that individuals are ready to act if they

    - Believe they are susceptible to the condition (i.e., perceived susceptibility)

    - Believe the condition has serious consequences (i.e., perceived severity)

    - Believe that taking action reduces their susceptibility to the condition or its severity (i.e., perceived benefits)

Self-Determination Theory

The underlying assumption of the ***self-determination theory (SDT)*** is that individuals have three primary psychosocial needs that they are trying to satisfy

- Self-determination or autonomy

- Demonstration of competence or mastery

- Relatedness or ability to experience meaningful social interactions with others

296   Chapter 15—Overweight, Obesity, and Weight Control

The theory proposes that motivation exists on a continuum from amotivation to intrinsic motivation, with amotivation having the lowest levels of self-determination and intrinsic motivation having the highest degree of self-determination.

THEORY OF PLANNED BEHAVIOR

- According to the ***theory of planned behavior (TPB)***, intention to perform a behavior is the primary determinant of actual behavior.

- Intentions reflect an individual's probability that they will exercise but do not always translate directly into behavior because of issues related to behavioral control.

- "I intended to go for a walk today, but........"

SOCIAL ECOLOGICAL

- Social ecological models are important because they consider the impact of and connections between individuals and their environments.

- The explicit recognition of relations between an individual and their physical environment is a defining feature of ecological models.

- Behavior results from influences at multiple levels, including intrapersonal factors, interpersonal/cultural factors, organizational factors, physical environments, and policies.

Decreasing Barriers to Physical Activity

Lack of time:

- Identify available time slots. Monitor your daily activities for 1 week. Identify at least 30 minute time slots you could use for physical activity.

- Add physical activity to your daily routine.

- Select activities that require minimal time, such as walking, jogging, or stair climbing.

- Discuss modifications to their exercise prescription (FITT principles).

- Examine priorities and goals.

Chapter 15—Overweight, Obesity, and Weight Control   297

Social Influence

- Explain your interest in physical activity to friends and family. Join groups such as YMCA.

- Develop social support structures to help address barriers such as daycare.

- Exercise with family members.

Lack of Energy

- Schedule physical activity for times in the day or week you feel energetic. Understand that energy levels will likely improve with exercise

- Discuss modifications to their exercise prescription (adjust exercise intensity as needed).

Lack of Motivation

- Plan ahead by writing activities in calendar.

- Look for social support from friends and family.

- Discuss attitudes and outcome expectations.

- Determine stage of change and provide tailored counseling.

- Discuss potentially effective reinforcements.

Fear of Injury

- Choose activities that involve minimum risk (walking).

- Learn how to warm up and cool down.

- Determine task-specific self-efficacy.

Lack of Resources

- Adjust exercise prescription to use types of exercise that require minimal facilities and equipment.

- Evaluate exercise opportunities in the environment.

Cognitive and Behavioral Strategies for Increasing Physical Activity

- Cognitive strategies focus on changing the way individuals think, reason, and imagine themselves in regard to exercise behavior.

- Behavioral strategies refer to individual actions and reactions to environmental stimuli. Because actions and reactions are thought to be learned, the behavioral approach suggests that these actions and reactions can be unlearned or modified.

- Cognitive and behavioral strategies include enhancing **self-efficacy**, **goal setting**, **reinforcement**, **social support**, **self-monitoring**, **problem solving**, and **relapse prevention**.

Enhancing self-efficacy

- Ensure goals are realistic.
- Use tasks the individual will be able to complete successfully.
- Watch others who are similar to them have positive experiences.
- Provide verbal encouragement.
- Discuss physiological feedback.

Goal setting

- Goal setting is a powerful tool for behavior change that cuts across numerous theories but must be done as part of an ongoing process to be effective.
- Set both short- and long-term goals. Individuals often focus on long-term goals; however when attempting a new behavior, setting achievable short-term goals is important for increasing self-efficacy.
- The SMARTS principle can be used to guide effective goal setting.
  - *Specific*:
  - *Measureable*:
  - *Action-oriented*:
  - *Realistic*:
  - *Timely*:
  - *Self-determined*:

Reinforcement

- Individuals should be encouraged to reward themselves for meeting behavioral goals.
- Extrinsic rewards include tangible, physical rewards (e.g., new pair of shoes) and social reinforcement (e.g., praise).
- Intrinsic rewards come from within, such as a feeling of accomplishment. Individuals are more likely to adhere to exercise over the long term if they are doing the activity for intrinsic reasons such as for fun, enjoyment, and challenge.
- It may be difficult to give intrinsic reinforcers to participants, but it may be possible to develop an environment that can promote intrinsic motivation.
- These environments focus on the autonomy of the participant and have been shown to lead to higher levels of physical activity.

Social support

Social support can be provided to clients/patients in various ways including:

- Guidance:
- Reliable alliance:
- Reassurance of worth:

- Attachment:

- Social integration:

- Opportunity for nurturance:

Self-monitoring

Self-monitoring involves observing and recording behavior and is important in exercise behavior change.

Self-monitoring can take many forms such as:

- Paper-and-pencil log

- Heart rate monitor

- Pedometer or wearable technology

Problem Solving

Problem solving assists individuals in identifying strategies to eliminate barriers and includes four main steps:

- Identify the barrier

- Brainstorm ways to overcome the barrier

- Select a strategy that is likely to be successful

- Analyze how well the plan worked and revise as necessary

Relapse Prevention

Active individual may encounter situations that make sticking to their exercise program difficult or nearly impossible. Relapse prevention can be implemented across all approaches once individuals adopt and try to maintain exercise.

Relapse prevention strategies include:

- Being aware of and anticipating high-risk situations (e.g., travel, vacation, holiday, illness, family obligations, inclement weather).

- Having a plan to ensure that a lapse does not become a relapse.

Strategies to Facilitate Stage of Change Transitions

PRECONTEMPLATION → CONTEMPLATION

- Provide information about the benefits of regular physical activity.

- Discuss how some of the barriers they perceive may be misconceived such as: "It can be done in shorter and accumulated bouts if they don't have the time".

- Have them visualize what they would feel like if they were physically active with an emphasis on short-term, easily achievable benefits of activity such as sleeping better, reducing stress, and having more energy.

- Explore how their inactivity impacts individuals other than themselves such as their spouse and children.

CONTEMPLATION → PREPARATION

- Explore potential solutions to their physical activity barriers.

- Assess level of self-efficacy and begin techniques to build efficacy.

- Emphasize the importance of even small steps in progressing toward being regularly active.

- Encourage viewing oneself as a healthy, physically active person.

PREPARATION → ACTION

- Help develop an appropriate plan of activity to meet their physical activity goals and use a goal setting worksheet or contract to make it a formal commitment.

- Use reinforcement to reward steps toward being active.

- Teach self-monitoring techniques such as tracking time and distance.

- Continue discussion of how to overcome any obstacles they feel are in their way of being active.

- Encourage them to help create an environment that helps remind them to be active.

- Encourage ways to substitute sedentary behavior with activity.

ACTION → MAINTENANCE

- Provide positive and contingent feedback on goal progress.

- Explore different types of activities they can do to avoid burnout.

- Encourage them to work with and even help others become more active.

- Discuss relapse prevention strategies.

- Discuss potential rewards that can be used to maintain motivation.

Special Populations

An important area of exercise promotion is the proper tailoring of interventions to promote exercise behavior across diverse populations that present unique challenges.

Proper tailoring requires an understanding of potential unique beliefs, values, environments, and obstacles within a population or individual.

Older Adults

- Older adults may lack knowledge about the benefits of PA or how to set up a safe and effective exercise program so health/fitness and clinical exercise professionals need to provide some initial education.

- Although typically viewed as beneficial, social support is not necessarily positive, especially in older adults.

Chapter 15—Overweight, Obesity, and Weight Control   301

- Family and friends may exert negative influences by telling them to "take it easy" and "let me do it."

- The implicit message is that they are too old or frail to be physically active.

- Many of the typical barriers to physical activity are similar among younger and older adults such as lack of time and motivation; however, there are several barriers that may take on special significance among older adults.

- These barriers include lack of social support and increased social isolation.

- Quite possibly, the largest barrier to exercise participation in older adults is the fear that exercise will cause injury, pain, and discomfort or exacerbate existing conditions.

Youth

- When working with children, it is important to recognize that they are likely engaging in an exercise program because their parents wish them to, implying an extrinsic motivation, and typically require tangible forms of social support (e.g., transportation, payment of fees).

- To help them maintain exercise behavior over their lifetime, children need help shifting toward a sense of autonomy and to feel a sense of self-efficacy and behavioral control.

- It is imperative to work toward establishing a sense of autonomy and intrinsic motivation through the creation of a supportive environment.

Individuals with Obesity

- Individuals with obesity may face unique weight-related barriers to exercise (e.g., feeling uncomfortable while exercising, being uncomfortable with their appearance).

- Individuals with obesity may have had negative mastery experiences with exercise in the past and will need to enhance their self-efficacy so that they will believe they can successfully exercise.

- They may also be quite deconditioned and perceive even moderate intensity exercise as challenging, so keeping activities fun and at a low enough intensity that they feel positive may be particularly important.

- Individuals with obesity may need help setting realistic weight loss goals and identifying appropriate levels of physical activity to help them reach those goals.

Review Questions for Chapter 15

(For true and false questions that are false, indicate what would make the question true)

1. True or False:

   Over the past 30 years, the primary cause of overweight and obesity in the United States is lack of physical activity because caloric expenditure has remained fairly stable.

2. List 10 complications (co-morbidities) associated with obesity.

3. Define overweight. Give the BMI standard:

4. Define obesity. Give the BMI standard:

5. State the First Law of Thermodynamics and briefly describe how it is related to body weight.

6. What makes up the largest portion of one's daily energy expenditure?

7. True or False: A person's genetics plays only a small (≤25%) role in body weight and the development of obesity.

Chapter 15—Overweight, Obesity, and Weight Control   303

8. The heritability estimate of BMI most closely resembles:
   a. Eye color

   b. Foot size

   c. Hair color

   d. Body height

   e. None of these

9. _____ is a hormone produced by the _____ which normally interacts with the brain to blunt the drive to eat.

   a. Adiponectin; adipose tissue

   b. Adiponectin; liver

   c. Leptin; adipose tissue

   d. Leptin; liver

   e. None of these

10. True or False:

    Most obese individuals have a mutation in their leptin gene and therefore do not produce enough of this hormone which is the way they gain weight

11. True or False:

    An excessive amount of uncoupling protein within the adipose tissue and skeletal muscle would result in a reduced BMR and therefore weight gain

12. True or False:

    Studies have clearly shown that it is better to be of ideal body weight but low fitness then to be fit but over weight.

13. List the criteria (standards) for excessive body fat.

14. Adipose tissue located in the _____ has been shown to be a risk factor for the metabolic syndrome.

    a. Abdominal area

    b. Thigh region

    c. Gluteal region

    d. Triceps area

    e. None of these

15. _____ is a rate-limiting enzyme that facilitates uptake and storage of triglyceride by fat cells.

16. List the three important times for fat cell development.

17. Childhood obesity is associated with _____ of fat cells while adult onset would be related to _____ of these cells.
    a. Hypertrophy; hyperplasia
    b. Hyperplasia; hypertrophy
    c. Atrophy; hypertrophy
    d. Hyperplasia; atrophy
    e. None of these

18. True or False:

    The goal of most weight loss programs is to have the individual attempt to lose 3 to 5 lb per week.

19. New recommendations are for obese individuals to reduce initial body weight by _____.

20. List four characteristics of individuals who have lost 10% or more of their body weight and have kept the weight off for at least one year.

21. Define the set-point theory.

22. True or False:

    The existent literature appears to provide little evidence that exercise alone is a potent strategy for weight loss.

23. It takes a deficit of approximately _____ kcal to lose one pound of fat.

24. True or False:

Exercise must be of moderate to vigorous intensity and done continuously for at least 45 minutes to be effective for weight loss.

25. Wrestlers should be encouraged not to go below _____ body fat during their competitive season.

a. 3–5%

b. 5–7%

c. 7–10%

d. 1–2%

e. There is no recommendation for this population

26. _____ refers to an individual's belief that she or he can actually do a particular behavior in question.

a. Self-Control

b. Task self-efficacy

c. Self-determination

d. Preparation

e. Barrier self-efficacy

27. Which behavioral theory indicates that one's beliefs about whether they are susceptible to disease and their perceptions of the benefits of trying to avoid it influence their readiness to act?

a. Social cognitive theory

b. Transtheoretical model

c. Health belief model

d. Self determination theory

e. Theory of planned behavioral

28. List in order, the 5 different stages of readiness of the transtheoretical model.

29. Which of these strategies could be utilized for the common exercise barrier "I don't have enough time"?

   a. Maintain a calendar to identify time slots for physical activity.

   b. Discuss physical activity guidelines and modifications to exercise prescription (FITT) principles.

   c. Find a friend who is willing to exercise as a partner.

   d. A and B

   e. A, B, and C are all correct

Chapters 14 & 15

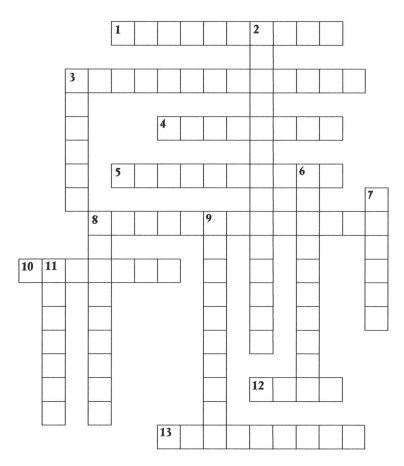

ACROSS

1 Technology that can assess the thickness of different tissues.

3 A number derived from body mass and stature used to assess normalcy for body weight.

4 Theory that states that all persons have a well-regulated internal control mechanism that maintains a preset body weight.

5 Includes fat primarily in adipose tissue.

8 Techniques used to quantify body size, proportion and shape.

10 A pincer type tool used to accurately mesure subcutaneous fat at selected anatomical sites.

12 Technology that can analyze regional body fat deposition.

13 Diet that emphasizes carbohydrate restriction while generally ignoring total calories, cholesterol and fat content.

DOWN

2 Irregular menstrual cycle.

3 Helium displacement plethysmography method to measure body volume.

6 The complete cessation of menses.

7 Fat deposition around the hips and buttocks.

8 Fat cell.

9 Refers to a body weight that exceeds some average for stature and age.

11 Fat deposition in the abdominal area.

Chapter 15—Overweight, Obesity, and Weight Control 309

Unit 3

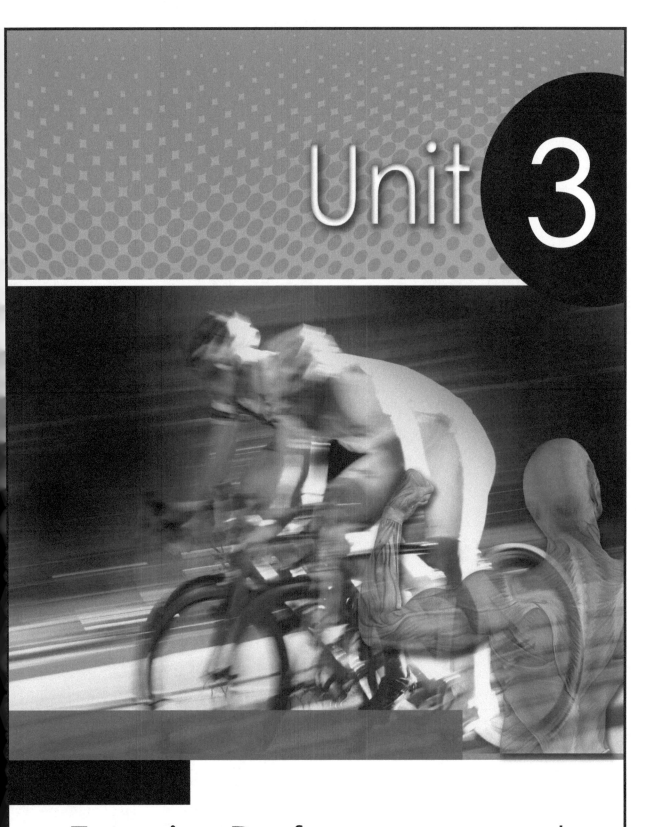

Exercise Performance and Environmental Stress

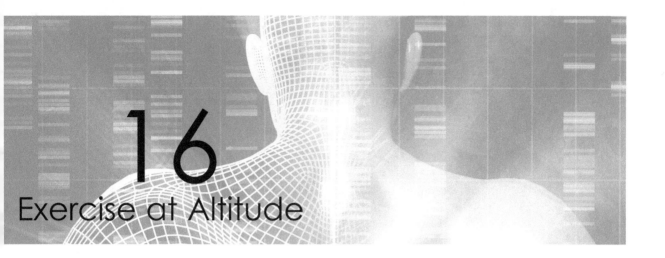

Exercise at Altitude

- Elevations 10,000 ft above sea level are considered *high altitude*
- Endurance exercise performance is reduced with increasing altitude (even as low as 4,000 and 5,000 ft)

How was performance affected in Mexico City during the 1968 Olympics?

- Events <400 m were _____
- Events >800 m were _____

Oxygen transport cascade is the progressive change in the environment's oxygen pressure and various body areas.

Altitude's physiologic challenge comes directly from decreased ambient P_{O_2}.

Fick's Law of Diffusion

Exchange of gases between the lungs and blood, and between blood and tissues, occurs passively (by diffusion) and is dependent on the pressure gradient.

Pressure is typically measured in mmHg (or torr) using what instrument? _____.

Atmospheric (barometric) pressue is (increased / unchanged / reduced) at altitude?

FIO_2 is (increased / unchanged / reduced) at altitude?

Arterial O_2 (PaO_2) is (increased / unchanged / reduced) at altitude?

Hemoglobin saturation (SaO_2) is (increased / unchanged / reduced) at altitude?

Effects of Hypoxia:

Respiratory alkalosis occurs due to hypoxic ventilatory drive (HVR)

- HVR is created by peripheral chemoreceptors.

The pressure gradient for O_2 diffusion is decreased with altitude, therefore reducing the driving pressure and increasing the time needed for diffusion.

Causes of Hypoxemia (Low Arterial PO_2):

1.

2.

3.

4.

5.

Performance at Altitude

Immediate Physiologic Response to Altitude:

a. Hyperventilation

- Hypoxia leads to increased ventilation (V_E), which leads to respiratory alkalosis.

- Central chemoreceptors in the brain sense the reduced $PaCO_2$ which ultimately leads to a reduced V_E.

b. Hypoxic pulmonary vasoconstriction (HPV)

- Increases resistance to blood flow through the lung

c. Increased HR and cardiac output

d. Increased catecholamines (i.e. Norepinephrine)

e. Increased fluid loss

- Dry environment, greater evaporation

f. Sensory function decreases

Short-Term Responses to Altitude (hours to days):

- Release of central inhibition (due to low $PaCO_2$) further increases ventilation

    After 1 to 3 days in hypoxia:

    - Choroid plexus excretes $HCO_3^- \Rightarrow$ CSF pH $\downarrow$ (to normal)

    - "Releases the brake" on ventilation, $\therefore \uparrow V_E$ further

- Erythropoiesis (increases hematocrit and hemoglobin)

- Decrease in plasma volume (increases hematocrit)

314   Chapter 16—Exercise at Altitude

Long-Term Adjustments to Altitude

- Cellular adaptations
  - Increased capillarization? Still controversial
    - Brain tissue—yes
    - Skeletal muscle—probably not without exercise
  - Increased 2,3 DiPhosphoGlycerate (DPG)
    - Shifts oxygen dissociation curve to the right
  - Increased mitochondrial density
  - Increased aerobic enzyme activities
- Loss of body weight (mostly lean body mass)
- Hypoxic desensitization (after many years, likely decades)

The adjustments to altitude are called:

- **Acclimatization**:

- **Acclimation**:

How long does acclimatization take?

Exercise and Training at Altitude

- Live-low and train-low (*do nothing and suffer!*)
- Live-low and train-high (lower absolute work levels)
- Live-high (acclimatize) and train-high (lower absolute work levels)
- Live-high (acclimatize) and train-low (high absolute work levels)
  - Thought to be best the physiologic approach to achieving maximum performance at altitude
  - Benefits of LHTL are controversial

- Essential for optimal exercise performance at altitude
- However, no benefit to aerobic capacity upon return to sea level!
- Possible negative effects of long-term high-altitude exposure:

Exercise and Lactate

There is a relationship between work and lactic acid/oxygen deficit.

Lactate is buffered by sodium bicarbonate:

$$La + NaHCO_3 \leftrightarrow NaLa + H_2CO_3$$

As lactate is buffered, CO_2 is regenerated from formation of carbonic acid thereby stimulating ventilation:

$$CO_2 + H_2O \leftrightarrow H_2CO_3 \leftrightarrow H^+ + HCO_3^-$$

Paradox:

- What is the lactate paradox?

- Mechanism for the lactate paradox:
  - Reduced glucose mobilization (via lower epinephrine)
  - Diminished intracellular ADP
  - Reduced CNS output
  - Carbon dioxide, retained through the Haldane effect, inhibits cellular excitation and sustaining oxidative metabolism to consume lactate efficiently

Medical Problems Related to Altitude:

- Acute mountain sickness
  - Due to hypoxia and respiratory alkalosis
- Chronic mountain sickness
  - Excessive polycythemia; symptoms include lethargy, weakness, sleep disturbances, cyanosis, decreased mental status
  - High-altitude pulmonary edema (HAPE)
  - High-altitude cerebral edema (HACE)

Hypoxic pulmonary vasoconstriction HPV increases pulmonary artery pressure

Uneven HPV is thought to contribute to development of HAPE

- High-altitude retinal hemorrhage (HARH)
  - Occurs in virtually all climbers above 22,000 ft (6,700 m)

17
Diving Depth and Pressure

- Water is noncompressible, so its pressure against a diver's body increases directly with the depth of the dive.

- Forces that produce hyperbaria in diving:

  - Weight of column of water directly above the diver

  - Weight of the atmosphere at the water's surface

- Good news: Water is a large portion of the body's tissues, so they are not susceptible to increased external pressure in diving.

- Bad news: Volume and pressure of the body's *air-filled cavities* alter greatly with any increase or decrease in diving depth, and death occurs if adjustments do not equal pressure changes.

- Boyle's law: At constant temperature, the volume of a given mass of gas varies inversely with its pressure.

  - When pressure doubles, volume halves; conversely, reducing pressure by one-half expands any gas volume to twice its previous size.

  - Failure to permit the extra air volume to escape through the nose or mouth during ascent allows the powerful force of expanding gases to rupture lung tissue.

Types of Diving

a. Snorkeling—A snorkel allows a swimmer to breathe continually with the face immersed in water.

   Limits to snorkel size:

   - Increased pulmonary dead space by enlarging the snorkel's volume

   - Increased hydrostatic pressure on the chest cavity as one descends beneath the water

b. Breath-hold diving

   - Most persons can breath-hold for up to 1 minute.

Chapter 17—Diving Depth and Pressure   317

- P_{O_2} drops to 60 mmHg and P_{CO_2} rises to 50 mmHg, signaling an urgency to breathe
- After about 30 seconds, the carbon dioxide level in arterial blood increases, causing the diver to sense the need to breathe and surface quickly
- Physical activity greatly reduces breath-holding time because oxygen consumption and carbon dioxide production increase with exercise intensity.
- Duration and depth of a breath-hold dive depend on:
  - Breath-hold duration until arterial carbon dioxide pressure reaches the breath-hold breakpoint
  - Relationship between a diver's TLC and RLV

Shallow-Water Blackout

- Hyperventilation lowers P_{CO_2} (up to 15 mmHg), extending breath-hold duration because it takes longer for P_{CO_2} to reach the level that stimulates ventilation.
- Hyperventilation *does not* result in a corresponding increase in arterial P_{O_2}. Blackout occurs when P_{O_2} levels are insufficient to maintain cerebral function.
- Other risks in hyperventilating before a breath-hold dive:
  - A normal quantity of arterial carbon dioxide maintains the blood's acid–base balance
  - Normal arterial P_{CO_2} stimulates dilation of arterioles in the brain

Diving Reflex in Humans

- Physiologic responses to immersion enable diving mammals to spend considerable time under water:
  - Bradycardia
  - Decreased cardiac output
  - Increased peripheral vasoconstriction
  - Lactate accumulation in underperfused muscle
  - Blood shift
    - Blood plasma fills up blood vessels in the lung, which reduces residual volume. Without this adaptation, the human lung would shrink and wrap into its walls causing permanent damage at depths greater than 30 m (98.4 ft).

c. Scuba diving

- Scuba (**s**elf-**c**ontained **u**nderwater **b**reathing **a**pparatus) is the most common apparatus for supplying air under pressure for complete independence from the surface.

318   Chapter 17—Diving Depth and Pressure

- The scuba system includes a tank of compressed air and a demand regulator valve that delivers air the diver needs at a particular depth with hose and mouthpiece or full face mask.
- Basic scuba designs:
  - Open-circuit system
  - Closed-circuit system

Special Problems with Breathing Gases at High Pressures:

- Scuba tanks supply air (or gas) at a pressure greater than force of water against the diver's thorax.
- If a diver takes a full breath at 10 m but fails to exhale while ascending, the rapidly expanding gas eventually ruptures the lungs before the diver reaches the surface.
- Air embolism from pulmonary barotrauma is second only to drowning as cause of death in recreational scuba divers.

Breath-Holding and Scuba Diving:

To eliminate the danger of air embolism and pneumothorax, divers need to ascend slowly and breathe normally when using scuba gear.

Pneumothorax (lung collapse):

- Air forced through the alveoli when lung tissue ruptures migrates laterally to burst through the pleural sac that covers the lungs.
- An air pocket forms in the chest cavity outside the lungs, between the chest wall and the lung.
- Continued expansion of trapped air during ascent collapses the ruptured lung.

Special Problems with Breathing Gases at High Pressures:

- Henry's Law: The quantity of gas dissolved in a liquid at a given temperature varies directly with the pressure differential between the gas and the liquid and the gas solubility in the liquid.
- The partial pressure of each gas in the breathing mixture increases; for example:
  - At 10 m (33 ft), the nitrogen partial pressure doubles the sea-level value to 1200 mmHg
  - 300 ft in sea water (fsw), or approximately 90 m, generally sets the limit for compressed-air diving, because dissolved nitrogen in the body's fluids and tissues renders most incapable of accomplishing meaningful work

Nitrogen narcosis:

- Narcosis, from *narke* (Greek origin), means "temporary decline or loss of senses and movement"

Chapter 17—Diving Depth and Pressure   319

- Divers experience increasing narcosis and mental impairment with increasing depth (resulting in impaired mental behavior that is similar to alcohol intoxication).

- Begins around 10 m (but is negligible); usually becomes noticeable at 30 m (approximately100 ft)

Oxygen toxicity:

- Inspiring a gas with a P_{O_2} above 2 ATA greatly increases a diver's susceptibility to oxygen poisoning, particularly at elevated metabolic rates during physical activity.

- Breathing high pressures of oxygen negatively affects bodily functions in three ways:

  - Irritates respiratory passages and eventually induces bronchopneumonia if exposure persists

  - Constricts cerebral blood vessels at pressures above 2 ata and alters central nervous system function

  - Depresses carbon dioxide elimination

Decompression sickness:

- Occurs when dissolved nitrogen moves out of solution and forms bubbles in body tissues and fluids

  - Results from ascending to the surface too rapidly following a deep, prolonged dive

  - Also known as the "bends"

- Treatment involves lengthy recompression in a hyperbaric chamber, which elevates external pressure to force nitrogen gas back into solution, and then slowly (gradually) decompressing, allowing time for the expanding gas to leave the body as the diver returns to the surface pressure.

  - Immediate recompression offers the best chance for success; any delay decreases the prognosis for complete recovery

d. Mixed-gas diving

- Three mixtures of oxygen, nitrogen, and helium are used for deep and saturation diving:

  - **Nitrox** (↓ nitrogen + ↑ oxygen): relatively shallow recreational dives

  - **Heliox** (helium + oxygen): deep diving

  - **Trimix** (helium + nitrogen + oxygen): dives to depths that may produce high-pressure nervous syndrome

- Technical divers (military, salvage, science) routinely use various **Trimix** (helium + nitrogen + oxygen) combinations:

  - Compressed gas to dive below 300 fsw, because blending a depth-specific gas mixture allows them to control the risk of hyperoxia and the narcotic potential of nitrogen

Other Diving-Related Problems:

- Mask squeeze
    - Periodically exhaling through the nose into the mask balances pressures on both sides of the face mask
- Middle ear squeeze (aerotitis)
    - In scuba diving, middle-ear pressure equalizes with external pressure by blowing gently against closed nostrils
- Sinus squeeze (aerosinusitis)
    - Inflamed, congested sinuses prevent air pressure in these cavities from equalizing during diving
    - Sinus air pressure that does not equalize during descent, remains at atmospheric pressure while external pressure increases
    - This relative vacuum creates "sinus squeeze," causing sinus membranes to bleed as blood occupies the space to equalize the pressure differential

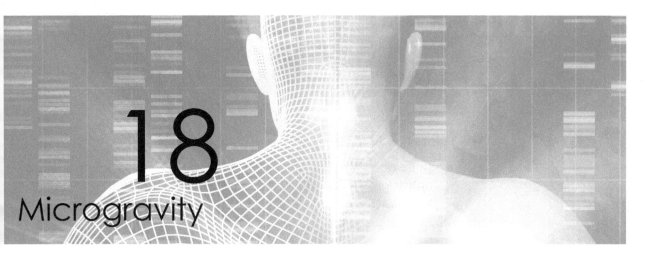

18
Microgravity

OUTER SPACE

The physiological challenges associated with exploration in outer space relate to zero pressure and microgravity. Three important physiologic effects occur in response to micrograity....

1. Fluid shifts
2. Unloading on weight-bearing structures
3. Metabolic changes

   - Microgravity results in loss of hydrostatic gradient
   - Blood and fluid volumes shift upward and move into the thoracocephalic region, causing:
     - A puffy-face appearance, a 2- to 5-cm decrease in the waist, eye redness, skinny legs, nasal congestion, headaches, and nausea
   - Blood volume, plasma volume, and red blood cell volume decrease
   - There is decrease venous pooling, blunted baroreceptor reflex, and orthostatic intolerance

Cardiovascular Adaptations in Microgravity:

- Cardiac output: _____
- Blood pressure: _____
- Cardiac Size: _____
- Decrease in total fluid volume reduces the heart's total work effort
- Decrease in total fluid volume helps to reduce the heart's total work effort
- These adaptations represent an appropriate response without compromising normal cardiovascular function
- Orthostatic intolerance (fainting) occurs upon return to Earth's gravity.

Chapter 18—Microgravity   323

Pulmonary Adaptations in Microgravity:

- Gas exchange is mostly unaltered with microgravity

  - Spaceship environments are maintained at **760 torr** (sea-level equivalent)

  - Residual volume and FRC decrease

- Pulmonary blood measures are all increased

  - Increased Q, increased pulmonary capillary blood volume, more uniform distribution of blood throughout the lung – but inequality still remains.

- Pulmonary ventilation is increased

  - Increased frequency and increased tidal volume, but alveolar ventilation is mostly unchanged

  - The distribution of ventilation is more even, though inequality still remains

Musculoskeletal Adaptations in Microgravity:

- NASA's greatest biomedical concern involves the 1% per month loss in weight-bearing bone mass during missions.

  - In a microgravity environment, reduced calcium intestinal absorption exacerbates calcium fecal loss

  - Even with on-board physical exercise intervention, bone loss persists and can remain pathologic for a prolonged period following a mission

  - Bone loss during prolonged microgravity exposure coincides with considerable decrements in muscle mass and strength

Muscle Ultrastructural Changes in Microgravity:

- Decreased aerobic enzyme activity

- Decreased muscle capillarity

- In-flight and post-flight changes during missions of nearly 1 year include:

  - Altered muscular coordination patterns

  - Delayed-onset muscle soreness

  - Generalized muscular fatigue and weakness

- Permanent neuromuscular dysfunction has not yet been demonstrated during prolonged space missions

Body Composition Changes in Microgravity:

- Minimal or no changes in body fat or extracellular water

- 2 to 3% decline in body mass attributable to a loss in fat-free mass (FFM)

- All three components of FFM (water, protein, and mineral) declined from 3 to 4% in post-flight measures

324   Chapter 18—Microgravity

Exercise as Countermeasure during Spaceflight

Countermeasure Strategies to Microgravity:

- Without appropriate countermeasures, microgravity's deleterious effects mimic the adverse changes of prolonged bed rest

  - Decrements in cardiovascular function generally parallel losses in muscle strength and size

- In-flight resistance and endurance exercises show the greatest overall potential as exercise countermeasures

Extravehicular Activity (EVA)—Space Walking

- Before EVAs, astronauts wash out nitrogen from their fluids and tissues (called denitrogenation) to minimize or prevent decompression sickness

  - A 10.2 lb psia staged decompression of the shuttle for at least 12 hours prior to EVA

  - 100 minutes of preoxygenation breathing 100% O_2 prior to EVA

- The rate of denitrogenation depends on:

  - Tissue nitrogen capacity, which increases with body fat content

  - Tissue oxygenation, which depends on cardiac output

Strategies to Simulate Microgravity

Strategies to simulate a microgravity environment and study its effects on humans include:

- Head-down bed rest

- Wheelchair confinement of paraplegics

- Immobilization and confinement

- Water immersion

- Parabolic flights

Simulating microgravity allows researchers to manipulate various experimental conditions before deciding on the best procedure for a particular mission:

- Test equipment that creates zero-g conditions for relatively brief times with nonhuman objects dropped from towers and into tubes

- Parabolic airplane flights with living and nonliving objects

- Head-down bed rest, confinement, water immersion, or immobilization

Space Pharmacology

- Space motion sickness (SMS) remains the most persistent short-term problem during space flight.

- To date, no single pharmacologic treatment prevents or cures SMS, due in part to incomplete understanding of the cause, though medication provides the most effective pharmacologic therapy

Chapter 18—Microgravity   325

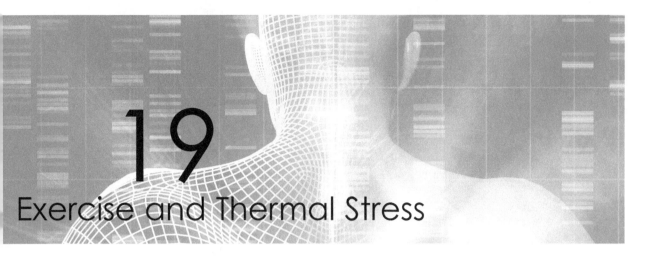

19
Exercise and Thermal Stress

Thermal Balance

1. The temperature of the body's inner tissues (known as the *core* temperature) is dependent on factors that add and/or subtract body heat. The general core temperature is therefore the balance between these two.
2. Several physiologic mechanisms are involved in the transfer of heat to the periphery, the loss of heat from the body, and the regulation of overall core body temperature.
3. Core temperature will rise if heat gain exceeds heat loss—something that often occurs during prolonged and intensive exercise.

Increased metabolic rate (increased energy metabolism) increases heat production:

- Shivering:
  - Exercise metabolism

Sweat rate can increase to 2.0 L/hour

Shivering can produce an oxygen consumption of approximately 1200 mL/min

Hypothalamus:

- Contains specialized neurons that coordinate and control temperature regulation of the body (acts as thermostat)

Regulates body temperature in two ways:

1.

2.

Peripheral Thermal Receptors

- Early warning system:
  - Sends sensory information to the hypothalamus and cortex
  - Evokes appropriate physiologic adjustments
- Free nerve endings in the skin
- Responsive to rapid changes in heat and cold
- Cold receptors:
  - More numerous
  - Exist near the skin surface
  - Initiate regulatory response to cold

Temperature of the Blood

- Changes in blood temperature detected by anterior hypothalamus
- Heightens activity and stimulates hypothalamus to initiate coordinated responses
- Posterior hypothalamus: heat conservation
- Anterior hypothalamus: heat loss

Review:

- Hypothalamus: _____ receptors in the skin provide input to the central control center. The more numerous _____ generally exist near the skin surface and evokes appropriate _____ mechanisms. Changes in the _____ of the blood that perfuses the _____ portion of the hypothalamus directly stimulates this area, causing a coordinated response for heat conservation from the _____ hypothalamus and heat dissipation from the _____ hypothalamus.

Heat Transfer

- Temperature gradient can flow from:
  - The body to the environment

    or

  - In extreme cold: increase heat production and minimize heat loss to prevent a decline in core temperature

Thermoregulation in Cold Stress

Vascular Adjustments:

- Stimulation of cutaneous cold receptors:
  1.
  2.
  3.

Average cutaneous blood flow rate is approximately 250 mL/min in a thermo-neutral environment; this can fall to approximately zero in environments that are extremely cold.

How might excessive body fat be beneficial in cold environments?

Muscular Activity:

- Exercise maintains a constant core temperature in air as cold as −30 °C
- Shivering: involuntary muscle contractions
- During exercise:
  - Shivering will occur during strenuous exercise if the core temperature remains low
  - When exercise stops and the metabolic rate of the individual falls, shivering may not be able to prevent a decline in core temperature
  - Muscle fatigue will not depress the shivering response

Hormonal Output:

Increased heat production occurs because of two "calorigenic" adrenal medulla hormones:

1.

2.

  - Prolonged Cold Exposure

The thermoregulation system protects primarily against overheating.

- During exercise in the heat, a competition exists between:
  1.
  2.
- There are four physical processes that facilitate heat loss:
  1. Radiation:
     - Consists of electromagnetic heat waves
     - Does not require molecular contact
     - The body is usually warmer than the environment
  2. Conduction:
     - Direct heat transfer requiring molecular contact
       - Through a solid, liquid, or gas
     - Heat moves through deep tissues to the cooler skin surface
     - Influenced by:
       a.
       b.

Chapter 19—Exercise and Thermal Stress   329

Conduction in Aquatic Environments:

- Water absorbs several thousand times more heat than air
- Water conducts heat away from the warmer body part
- Lose more heat in water (compared to air of same temperature)

Convection:

- Loss of heat due to movement of air or water adjacent to the skin
- Air passing from riding a bike accelerates heat loss
- Little air movement or convection creates a zone of insulation
  - Minimizes further conductive heat loss

Air flowing over the body produces a cooling effect, which forms the basis of the wind chill temperature index.

Evaporation:

- Heat loss via water vaporizing from the respiratory passages and skin surface
- 580 kcal of heat are lost per liter of water vaporized
- Evaporation and sweating
  - During heat stress, eccrine sweat glands secrete large quantities of hypotonic saline solution
  - Evaporation of sweat from the skin creates a cooling effect
  - The cooled skin in turn cools the blood diverted from interior tissues to the surface
- Evaporative cooling provides the body with the best defense against overheating.
- Evaporation from skin and pulmonary surfaces is influenced by:
  1.
  2.
  3.

When ambient temperature exceeds body temperature, the effectiveness of conduction, convection, and radiation is reduced. In this case, evaporative cooling is the only effective method. Relative humidity is the most important factor determining how well evaporative cooling functions.

Integration of Heat-Dissipating Mechanisms:

The physiological mechanisms that regulate heat loss are the same regardless of whether the heat load is coming from internal or external means.

330   Chapter 19—Exercise and Thermal Stress

The circulatory system is the main physiological system maintaining thermal balance.

- With extreme heat:

  •

- Sweating starts within several seconds of the start of vigorous exercise.

  •

- Increased heart rate:

  •

Hormonal Adjustments:

As sweating increases, both water (plasma) and electrolytes are lost, which causes specific hormones to be released.

Hormonal adjustments are stimulated by:

- •

- •

The magnitude of hormonal adjustments depends on the severity of hypohydration and the intensity of physical activity.

Aldosterone:

Vasopressin:

Effects of Clothing on Thermoregulation

- Reduces radiant heat gain in warm environments and helps prevent conductive and convective heat loss in the cold.

Clo Unit:

- Developed by military:
  - to develop standards for the insulative properties of clothing
  - to meet environmental challenges
- An index of thermal resistance
- Indicates the insulating capacity of any layer of air trapped between skin and clothing
- A clo unit of 1 maintains a sedentary person at 1 MET indefinitely in an environment of 21°C and 50% humidity
- Clo units needed are influenced by:

Ideal Clothing:

1. Cold
   - Several layers of light clothing lined with various materials often provide the best benefits.

Chapter 19—Exercise and Thermal Stress   331

- Blocks air movement
- Allows water vapor from sweating to escape
- Saturation of a garment affects heat exchange

2. Heat
   - Moist clothing is more effective in allowing evaporative heat loss.
     - Cottons and linens to absorb moisture
   - Football uniforms are limited in regard to heat exchange:

Exercise in the Heat

- There are two competing demands when one exercises in the heat:
  1.
  2.

Cardiac Output:

- Submaximal exercise:

- Maximal exercise:

  - *Higher* heart rates at *all* submaximal levels of exercise in the heat

    - This increase *does not* offset decreased SV

Compensatory Vasoconstriction:

- There is a compensatory vasoconstriction in splanchnic and renal vascular beds:
  a.
  b.
  c.

Maintenance of Blood Pressure:

- Visceral vasoconstriction increases total vascular resistance
- Intense exercise with accompanying dehydration:

Temperature regulation is compromised in order to maintain blood pressure (general circulation) and muscle blood.

Exertional Heat Stress:

- Greater dependence on *anaerobic* metabolism compared to cooler conditions

  -
  -
  -

- Exercising in the heat results in increased lactate accumulation

  -
  -

Core Temperature during Exercise:

- In environments where thermoregulatory mechanisms are inadequate:

- Fatigue often is associated with temperatures that range between 38 and 40 °C because of:
  - Higher brain temperatures decreasing central drive to exercise
  - Impaired muscle activation/depressed neuromuscular drive
  - Depressed GI blood flow and increased permeability of toxins (contribute to fatigue)

Relative workload (i.e., percentage of exercise capacity) determines change in core temperature with exercise.

Both trained and untrained have the same core temperature at any given %$\dot{V}O_2$ (relative)

-
-

Water Loss in the Heat—Dehydration:

- The sweat loss for moderate-intensity exercise lasting more than an hour is between 0.5 and 1.0 L
- Fluid deficits:

  -
  -

- Exercising in a dehydrated state increases the risk of heat illness
- Sweat remains hypotonic to other body fluids
- Loss of body water impairs exercise events that take longer than 1 min

Chapter 19—Exercise and Thermal Stress   333

- CV function and exercise capacity are compromised in hot environments (almost any level of dehydration can compromise performance and the ability to maintain thermal balance)
- Acclimatized individuals can lose water at a rate of approximately 3 L per hour through sweating
- Elite marathon runners have been reported to lose as much as 5 L during the competition; this would be equivalent to 6 to 10% of body mass
- For each liter of fluid lost through sweating, exercise HR increases approximately 8 beats per min.

Physiological Consequences of Fluid Loss:

1.

2.

3.

4.

5.

Fluid Balance

- Fluid replacement:

  -

  -

- The goal is to prevent dehydration:

  -

  -

- A well-hydrated athlete always functions at a higher level than one who exercises in a dehydrated state.

Hyperhydration:

- Delays hypohydration from inadequate fluid replacement

  -

- Increases sweating during exercise
- Produces smaller rise in core temperature
- Cold beverage before exercise in the heat:

  -

  -

  -

- Pure water dilutes plasma sodium
- Decreased plasma osmolality:

  -

  -

Recommendations for hyperhydration:

1. 500 mL the night before exercise
2. 500 mL in the morning
3. 400 to 600 mL of cold water before exercise

Electrolyte Replacement:

- Added sodium or potassium:

    -

- ACSM recommendations:

    -

- Maintaining a relatively high plasma sodium concentration by adding sodium to ingested fluid:

    -

    -

    -

Optimizing Hydration:

- Pre-exercise

    - Approximately 17 to 20 ounces, 2 to 3 hours before activity

    - Consume another 7 to 10 ounces after the warm-up (10 to 15 min before exercise)

- During exercise

    - Approximately 28 to 40 ounces every hour of exercise (7 to 10 ounces every 10 to 15 min)

    - Rapidly replace lost fluids (sweat and urine) within 2 hours after activity to enhance recovery by drinking 20 to 24 ounces for every pound of body weight lost through sweating

Five Factors Modify Heat Tolerance:

1.
2.
3.
4.
5.

Acclimatization:

- Heat acclimatization:

    - The collective physiologic adaptive changes that improve heat tolerance

- Major acclimatization occurs in the first week:

Chapter 19—Exercise and Thermal Stress   335

Physiologic adjustments during heat acclimatization response effect:

Improved cutaneous blood flow:	Transport metabolic heat from core to shell
Effective distribution of CO:	Appropriate circulation to skin and muscles to meet needs; greater BP stability
Lowered threshold for start of sweating:	Evaporative cooling begins early in exercise
More effective distribution of sweat over skin surface:	Optimum use of effective body surface for evaporative cooling
Increased sweat output:	Maximizes evaporative cooling
Lowered salt concentrations of sweat:	Preserves electrolytes in EC fluid
Lowered skin and core temperatures:	Greater proportion of CO to muscles
HR for standard exercise:	
Less reliance on CHO metabolism:	CHO sparing

Training adaptations facilitate elimination of metabolic heat generated by exercise

People who are well trained respond more effectively to sudden, severe heat stress.

Age:

- When controlled for body size and composition, there seems to be very little or no age-related decreases in thermoregulatory capacity or the ability to acclimatize to heat stress.
- Aging delays the onset of sweating and blunts the magnitude of the sweat response:
    -
    -
    -
- Decreased peripheral vascular sensitivity impairs local cutaneous vasodilation.

Children:

- Show a lower sweat rate and a higher core temperature
- Exercise intensity should decrease for children exposed to heat
- Require a longer time frame for heat acclimatization

Gender:

- Both genders acclimatize to the same degree
- Women tolerate thermal stress of exercise at least as well as men of comparable aerobic fitness and level of acclimatization

336   Chapter 19—Exercise and Thermal Stress

- Heat dissipation in women:

- Men make greater use of evaporative cooling

Body Fat Level:
- Fatal heat stroke occurs 3.5 times more frequently in obese young adults

Heat Stress Complications:
a. Heat cramps:

b. Heat exhaustion:
   - Ineffective circulatory adjustments
   - Blood pools in the dilated vessels
   - Characteristics of:

c. Heat stroke:
   - Requires immediate medical attention
   - Produces several problems:

   - Exertional heat stroke is a condition of extreme hyperthermia because of:
      1.
      2.

Exercise in the Cold
- Water conducts heat about 25 times faster than air
- The body is able to use different fuels effectively during sustained cold exposure

Body Fat, Exercise, and Cold Stress:
- Increased body fat retards heat loss
- Athletes with greater thermal insulation swim in cool ocean water with almost no decline in core temperature
   -
- Cold stress is highly relative

Children and Cold Stress:

Humans possess much less capacity for adaptation to long-term cold exposure than to prolonged heat exposure; must rely on external relief.

Ama:

- Female divers in Korea and southern Japan
- 45 min in summer (77 °F), only 15 min in winter (50 °F)
- Elevated resting metabolism may allow ama to tolerate colder temperatures

Wind Chill Temperature Index:

- Provides a useful way to understand the dangers from winter winds and freezing temperatures
- Air currents on a windy day magnify heat loss

Unit Three Review Questions

Name: _____

(For true and false questions that are false, indicate what would make the question true)

1. List the similarities and differences between the hypothalamus and a thermostat.

2. _____ are responsive to rapid changes in hot and cold. Changes in blood temperature are detected by the _____. The _____ hypothalamus is responsible for heat conservation and the _____ hypothalamus is responsible for heat loss.

3. True/False:

    General muscle fatigue will not depress the shivering response.

4. Which of the following influence conduction?

    a. State of the molecules (solid, liquid, gas)

    b. Temperature gradient

    c. Thermal qualities of the surface

    d. The windchill effect

    e. Relative humidity

5. How does humidity affect evaporation?

6. What happens to heart rate when stroke volume decreases at max exercise in the heat?

7. Which of the following occurs with heat stress and submaximal exercise?

    a. Earlier accumulation of lactate

    b. Less dependence on anaerobic metabolism

    c. Increased muscle catabolism of lactate

    d. Sustained endurance during prolonged exercise

Unit 3: Exercise Performance and Environmental Stress   339

8. While exercising in the heat, in the competition between the periphery, for temperature regulation, and the muscles, for energy and O_2 delivery, which side wins and why?

9. When core temperature exceeds 38 °C (100 °F), there is a _____ central drive to exercise, _____ muscle activation, _____ neuromuscular drive, and _____ GI blood flow, which allows _____ permeability of toxins that contribute to fatigue.

10. With endurance exercise in the heat, why does drinking a high-sodium beverage help?

11. What is the effect of the following adaptations to exercise in the heat?

   a. Sweating over more body surface area: _____

   b. More dilute sweat: _____

   c. Lower skin and core temperatures and HR for submax exercise: _____

12. True/False:

   Well-trained individuals respond more effectively to sudden, severe heat stress.

13. Which of the following are true of heat dissipation in women (compared to men)?

   a. Women sweat at lower skin and core temperatures

   b. Women sweat less prolifically

   c. Women lose heat more easily due to a higher ratio of surface area to volume

   d. Women make greater use of evaporative cooling mechanisms

14. Explain how excess body fat can be both beneficial and detrimental depending on the athlete.

15. Who can generate a higher metabolism?

   a. Untrained

   b. Elite strength athletes

   c. Elite endurance athletes

   d. This is independent of training

16. The primary concern with exercising at altitude is a reduced
_____.

17. True/False:

    The saturation of hemoglobin is greater at altitude, which makes it harder for oxygen to dissociate and therefore be available to the tissues.

18. Define hypoxia.

19. Define hypoxemia.

20. List three *immediate* physiological responses to altitude exposure.

21. List three *long-term* physiologic adjustments to altitude exposure.

22. It usually takes approximately how long to see significant acclimatization to an altitude of 2300 m or greater?
    a. One day
    b. One week
    c. Two weeks
    d. One month
    e. Three months

23. Briefly explain the concept "Live-High, Train-Low." Is this strategy effective?

24. True/False:

    Maximal work at high altitude by acclimatized individuals results in higher lactate production compared to maximal work done at sea level.

25. List five physiologic consequences of acute mountain sickness.

Unit 3: Exercise Performance and Environmental Stress   341

26. List four signs and symptoms of chronic mountain sickness.

27. True/False:

The biggest physiologic concern with diving occurs on the ascent, because as one comes closer to the surface, the lung volume decreases

28. True/False:

Snorkeling increases the dead space air of the swimmer.

29. Briefly discuss how physical activity affects breath-hold diving.

30. List three physiologic responses to immersion that enable certain mammals to stay under water for extended periods of time.

31. Define nitrogen narcosis and briefly explain how it occurs.

32. True/False:

Breathing high pressures of oxygen greatly increases the body's ability to eliminate carbon dioxide.

33. True/False:

The "bends" is caused by excess retention of carbon dioxide in a diver who ascends too quickly.

34. True/False:

During periods of microgravity, blood and fluid volumes shift upward and move into the thoracocephalic region, causing a puffy-face appearance.

35. Pulmonary adaptations in microgravity include:

   a. Increased cardiac output

   b. Increased pulmonary capillary blood volume

   c. Reduced tidal volume

   d. a and b

   e. All of these

36. Musculoskeletal adaptations in microgravity include:

a. Bone loss

b. Reduction in percentage of type I muscle fibers

c. Decreased muscle capillarity

d. a and b

e. All of these

Unit 4

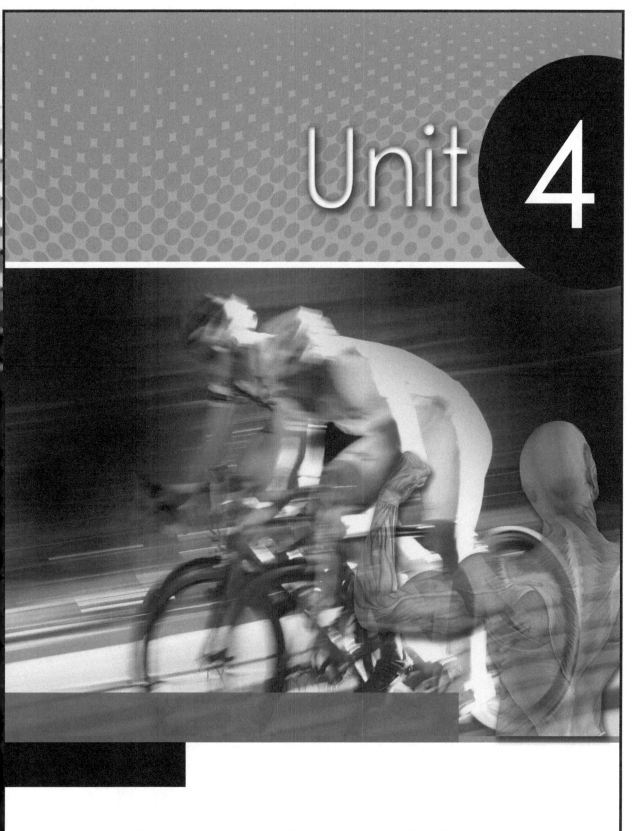

Exercise is Medicine

20
Electrocardiogram/Exercise for Rehabilitation

Single-lead electrocardiogram (ECG) provides a single view of the heart. A 12- lead ECG provides 12 short strips, allowing for multiple views of the heart.

Biphasic Deflection

- A biphasic deflection is one in which the deflection is equally positive and negative. This is produced when the electrical current is moving perpendicular to the positive electrode.

Negative Deflection

Positive Deflection

Limb Leads

- The combination of leads placed on the actual limbs of the body during a "Resting ECG" combine to give the ECG technician six different views of the heart.

Chapter 20—Electrocardiogram/Exercise for Rehabilitation   347

- Three bipolar (between two electrodes) views and 3 unipolar (from a central point in the heart outward) views
- **Lead I** = Right Arm (RA) – Left Arm (LA)
- **Lead II** = RA – LL
- **Lead III** = LA – LL

Unipolar Limb Leads

- These "augmented voltages" (aV) are labeled for the electrode that they look towards from the center of the heart.
- **aVR** = right
- **aVL** = left
- **aVF** = foot

Precordial "Chest" Leads

The Precordial "Chest" Leads view the heart along the horizontal plane.

- Bisects the heart into top and bottom halves
- V1 is effective in viewing the atria and intraventricular septum. Important in the determination of bundle branch block
- V2, V3, and V4 monitor the anterior wall of the left ventricle
- V5 and V6 view the lower left, lateral wall of the heart

Analysis Format for 12-Lead ECG

- Rhythm
- Axis deviation
- Bundle branch block
- Ischemia and infarction (remember paired leads)
- Chamber enlargement
- Miscellaneous changes

Axis Deviation of the Heart

Changing the angle of the heart can change the force vector. Increased muscle mass in the different chambers of the heart can also change the force vectors. The more muscle mass a chamber has, the more the force vector is directed to that area

- The normal angulation of the heart is downward and slightly angled to the left
- Because the left ventricle is the largest chamber, it naturally produces the most force

348   Chapter 20—Electrocardiogram/Exercise for Rehabilitation

CLINICAL EXERCISE TESTING

Graded exercise tests (GXT) are often used clinically to assess an individual's ability to tolerate increasing intensities of aerobic exercise.

Often the GXT is combined with the use of ECG, hemodynamic, and gas exchange measures to aid in the identification of suspected limitations. Under these situations the GXT is commonly referred to as a cardiopulmonary exercise test (CPET).

Reasons to perform CPET:

- Diagnostic

- Disease prognosis

- Therapeutic intervention effectiveness

- Transplant evaluation

- Exercise prescription

Patients with a high probability of disease (e.g., typical angina, prior coronary revascularization, or myocardial infarction) perform CPET:

- To assess residual myocardial ischemia

- To assess threatening ventricular arrhythmias

- For prognosis rather than for diagnostic purposes

CPET FOR DISEASE SEVERITY AND PROGNOSIS

The severity of coronary artery disease and resulting ischemia during CPET is often said to be:

- Proportional to the magnitude of ST-segment depression on ECG

- Proportional to the number of leads showing ST-segment abnormalities on the ECG

- Proportional to the duration of ST-segment depression into recovery

- Inversely proportional to the ST slope, the rate pressure product (RPP) at which the ST-segment depression occurs, and the heart rate maximum, SBP, and metabolic equivalents achieved

CPET AFTER HEART ATTACK (MYOCARDIAL INFARCTION)

Following a myocardial infarction, a CPET may be performed before hospital discharge for prognostic purposes as well as determining physical activity limitations (exercise prescription). However, this is usually not the case since many cardiac patients will be entering a Phase II cardiac rehabilitation program which will provide monitoring of hemodynamic responses to physical activity.

TYPES OF CPET

Two most common types of exercise modes utilized during CPET are the cycle ergometer and the motorized treadmill. In general, the mode of CPET should be individualized based upon the subjects' physical and health condition as well as the measurements that will be collected.

Cycle Ergometer Testing

- Lower VO_2max (5 to 25%)

- More accurate determination of work rate (Work = Force × Distance)

Motorized Treadmill Testing

- Higher VO_2max

- More common to most people

- More difficult to perform most measurements

- More likely to obtain true maximal effort

COMMON GXT PROTOCOLS

- Bruce
- Ellestadt
- Naughton
- Balke-Ware
- Ramp

MEASUREMENTS BEFORE, DURING, AND AFTER CPET

	Before CPET	During CPET	After CPET
ECG	Monitor cont. Record supine and standing	Monitor cont. Record last 15 sec/stage	Monitor cont.
HR	Monitor cont. Record supine and standing	Monitor cont. Record last 5 sec/min	Monitor cont.
BP	Measure and record supine/standing		
Signs/Symptoms	Monitor cont. Record as observed	Monitor cont. Record as observed	Monitor cont.
Perceived Exertion			
Gas Exchange			

INDICATIONS FOR TERMINATING CPET

- Absolute Indications

  1. Drop in systolic BP > 10 mmHg from baseline BP despite an increase in workload when in the presence of other evidence of ischemia
  2. Moderately severe angina
  3. Increasing nervous system symptoms (ataxia, dizziness)
  4. Poor perfusion
  5. Difficulties monitoring ECG or BP
  6. Subject's desire to stop
  7. Sustained V-Tach
  8. ST elevation (+1.0 mm) in leads without diagnostic Q-waves (other than V1 or aVR)

Chapter 20—Electrocardiogram/Exercise for Rehabilitation   351

- Relative Indications
  1. Drop in systolic BP of $\geq$10 mmHg with an increase in work rate, or if systolic BP below the value obtained in the same position prior to testing
  2. ST or QRS changes such as excessive ST depression (>2 mm horizontal or downsloping ST-segment depression) or marked axis shift
  3. Arrhythmias other than sustained ventricular tachycardia, including multifocal premature ventricular contractions (PVCs), triplets of PVCs, supraventricular tachycardia, heart block, or bradyarrhythmias
  4. Fatigue, shortness of breath, wheezing, leg cramps, or claudication
  5. Development of bundle branch block or intraventricular conduction delay that cannot be distinguished from ventricular tachycardia
  6. Increasing chest pain
  7. Hypertensive response (SBP of >250 mm Hg and/or a DBP of > 115 mm Hg).

Ecg, Cardiorespiratory, and Hemodynamic Responses to Cpet and their Clinical Significance

ST-Segment Depression

- ST-segment depression (depression of the J point and the slope at 80 msec past the J point) is the most common manifestation of exercise-induced myocardial ischemia.

- Horizontal or downsloping ST-segment depression is more indicative of myocardial ischemia than is upsloping depression.

- The standard criterion for a positive test is $\geq$1.0 mm (0.1 mV) of horizontal or downsloping ST segment at the J point extending for 60 to 80 msec.

- Slowly upsloping ST-segment depression should be considered a borderline response, and added emphasis should be placed on other clinical and exercise variables

- ST-segment depression does not localize ischemia to a specific area of myocardium

- The more leads with (apparent) ischemic ST-segment shifts, the more severe the disease

- Significant ST-segment depression occurring only in recovery likely represents a true positive response, and should be considered an important diagnostic finding.

- In the presence of baseline ST abnormalities $\geq$1.0 mm on the resting ECG, additional ST-segment depression during exercise is less specific for myocardial ischemia.

ST-Segment Elevation

- ST-segment elevation (early repolarization) may be seen in the normal resting ECG. Increasing HR usually causes these elevated ST segments to return to the isoelectric line.

- Exercise-induced ST-segment elevation in leads with Q waves consistent with a prior myocardial infarction may be indicative of wall motion abnormalities, ischemia, or both.
- Exercise-induced ST-segment elevation on an otherwise normal ECG (except in aVR or V_{1-2}) generally indicates significant myocardial ischemia, and localizes the ischemia to a specific area of myocardium. This response may also be associated with ventricular arrhythmias and myocardial injury.

Supraventricular Dysrhythmias

- Atrial arrhythmias and short runs of SVT often occur during CPET and do not appear to have any diagnostic or prognostic significance for CVD

Ventricular Dysrhythmias

- Suppression of resting arrhythmias with exercise does not exclude CVD
- Conversely, PVCs that increase in frequency, complexity, or both do not necessarily signify underlying ischemic heart disease
- Complex ventricular ectopy, including paired or multiform PVCs, and runs of ventricular tachycardia (≥3 successive beats) are likely to be associated with significant CVD and/or a poor prognosis if they occur in conjunction with signs and/or symptoms of myocardial ischemia in patients with a history of sudden cardiac death, cardiomyopathy, or valvular heart disease
- Frequent ventricular ectopy during recovery has been found to be a better predictor of mortality than ventricular ectopy that occurs only during exercise

HR

- The normal HR response to progressive exercise is a relatively linear increase, corresponding to 10 ± 2 beats $\cdot$ MET^{-1} for physically inactive subjects. Chronotropic incompetence may be signified by the following:
  - A peak exercise HR that is >2 SD (approximately 20 beats $\cdot$ min^{-1}) below the age-predicted HR$_{max}$ or an inability to achieve ≥85% of

the age-predicted HR_{max} for subjects who are limited by volitional fatigue and are not taking beta blockers

- A chronotropic index (CI) <0.8 (35); where CI is calculated as the ratio of heart rate reserve (HRR) to metabolic reserve achieved at any test stage

Recovery HR

- An abnormal (slowed) HR recovery is associated with a poor prognosis. Abnormal HR recovery has frequently been defined as a decrease ≤ 12 beats $\cdot$ min^{-1} at 1 min (walking in recovery), or ≤ 22 beats $\cdot$ min^{-1} at 2 min (supine position in recovery).

Systolic BP

- Progressive increase (10 mm Hg / MET) in SBP with a possible plateau at peak exercise. Terminate (relative indication for termination) exercise testing SBP > 250 mmHg.

- Exertional hypotension (SBP that fails to rise or falls [>10 mmHg]) may signify myocardial ischemia and/or LV dysfunction

- Maximal exercise SBP of <140 mmHg suggests a poor prognosis

Diastolic BP

- Normal response is no change or a decrease in DBP. A DBP of >115 mmHg is point for test termination relative indication.

Anginal Symptoms

- A rating of 3 (moderately severe) should be used as an endpoint for exercise testing absolute indication.

Interpreting Cpet

V_{O_2} and Work Rate.

- The V_{O_2} work rate relation describes how much O_2 is utilized in relation to the quantity of external work performed.

- In healthy subjects, steps at 1-minute increments provide smooth increases in V_{O_2} thereby allowing the slope of increase in V_{O_2} as a function of work rate to be calculated.

HR–Vo$_2$ and HRR

In healthy individuals, cardiac output and HR increase linearly with Vo$_2$ during incremental work. The slope of the HR–Vo$_2$ relationship is a function of SV and therefore cardiac function.

- In many types of heart diseases, the slope is steeper than normal and not as linear.

- COPD: Slope is steeper than normal (either decreased venous return to LV [hyperinflation] or deconditioning). Max HR is usually decreased in pulmonary patient.

- Maximal Heart Rate Reserve (HRR): The difference between predicted max HR, based on age, and the measured heart rate at peak Vo$_2$. Normally, maximal HRR is HRR is relatively small (less than 15 bpm).

O$_2$ Pulse

Remember: Vo$_2$ = HR × SV × a–Vo$_2$ difference. O$_2$ pulse = Vo$_2$/HR and therefore represents the O$_2$ extracted per heart beat.

- Often referred to as the "Poor man's SV"

Ventilatory Reserve and Capacity

Ventilatory reserve represents the relationship between ventilatory demand and ventilatory capacity (how close peak minute ventilation during exercise approaches MVV).

- $[(MVV-V_E \text{ peak})/(MVV \times 100)]$ or $[(V_E \text{ peak} / MVV) \times 100]$
- Healthy individuals: $V_{E \text{ peak}}$ during exercise approximately 70% of MVV
- Primary lung disease with ventilatory limitation to exercise = low breathing reserve

- Cardiovascular limitation to exercise = high breathing reserve

Exercise Prescription For Patients With CVD

Forms of Cardiovascular Disease

- Acute coronary syndromes:

- Cardiovascular disease:

- Cerebrovascular disease (stroke):

- CAD:

- Myocardial ischemia:

[ ]

- MI:

[ ]

- Peripheral arterial disease (PAD):

[ ]

Goals for Inpatient Rehabilitation

- Offset effects of bed rest.

- Provide additional medical surveillance.

- Identify patients with impairments influencing prognosis

[ ]

When to Discontinue Inpatient Exercise

- DBP ≥ 110 mmHg

- Decrease SBP > 10 mmHg during exercise

- Significant ventricular or atrial arrhythmias with or without associated signs/symptoms

- Second- or third-degree heart block

- Signs/symptoms of exercise intolerance including angina, marked dyspnea, and ECG changes suggestive of ischemia

Exercise Prescription for Inpatient

Frequency: Early mobilization with 2 to 4 times/day for first 3 days of hospital stay.

Intensity: Seated or standing resting HR + 20 bpm for those with an MI and +30 bpm for patients recovering from heart surgery; with an upper limit ≤ 120 bpm with a corresponding RPE ≤ 13 on a 6–20 scale.

Time: Intermittent walking bouts lasting 3 to 5 minutes as tolerated. Attempt to achieve a 2:1 exercise : rest ratio.

Type: Walking

Progression:

| |
| |

Exercise Prescription for Outpatient Program

Frequency: At least 3 days per week but preferably on most days of the week. For patients with very limited capacities, multiple short (1 to 10 minutes) daily sessions work best.

Intensity:

Based on results from the baseline exercise test, 40%–80% of exercise capacity using the HR reserve (HRR), oxygen uptake reserve (VO_2R), or peak oxygen uptake (VO_2peak) methods.

RPE of 11–16 on a scale of 6–20.

Exercise intensity should be prescribed at a HR below the ischemic threshold; for example, <10 beats, if such a threshold has been determined for the patient. The presence of classic angina pectoris that is induced with exercise and relieved with rest or nitroglycerin is sufficient evidence for the presence of myocardial ischemia.

Time: Warm-up and cool down activities of 5 to 10 minutes. Aerobic conditioning phase should be between 20 and 60 minutes per session.

Type: Aerobic portion should consist of rhythmic, large muscle group activities with an emphasis on increased caloric expenditure. Conditioning should include activities that use both upper and lower extremities.

Progression: Individualized based upon patient goals and tolerance.

ARTHRITIS

Arthritis is the leading cause of pain and disability in the United States. Of the adult US population, 22.2% (49.9 million) report having a doctor's diagnosis of arthritis. Two most common type of arthritis are **osteoarthritis** and **rheumatoid** arthritis.

- Osteoarthritis: is a local degenerative joint disease that can affect one or multiple joints.

- Rheumatoid: is a chronic, systemic inflammatory disease in which there is pathological activity of the immune system against joint tissue.

Exercise Testing and Arthritis

Most individuals with arthritis tolerate symptom limited graded exercise testing. Certain considerations should be noted.

- High-intensity exercise is contraindicated when there is acute inflammation. If individuals are experiencing acute inflammation, exercise testing should be postponed until the flare has subsided.

- The use of a cycle ergometer, with or without the use of the upper extremities, may be less painful than treadmill walking, and allow better assessment of cardiorespiratory function.

Exercise Prescription for Individuals with Arthritis

Frequency: Aerobic exercise 3 to 5 days per week, resistance exercise 2 to 3 days per week, flexibility should be performed daily.

Intensity: Light- to moderate-intensity physical activities are recommended because they are associated with lower risk of injury or pain exacerbation.

Time: Start with short bouts of 10 minutes progressing towards a goal of ≥150 minutes per week of aerobic exercise.

Type: Aerobic activities that are low impact are recommended whereas high-impact activities such as running, stair climbing, and those with stop and go actions should be avoided. Resistance and flexibility exercises should include all major muscle groups.

Progression: Progression should be gradual and individualized based upon pain and other symptoms.

Special Considerations for Those with Arthritis

- During acute inflammation, it is appropriate to gently move joints through full ROM.

- 5- to 10- minute warm up and cool down periods are critical for minimizing pain.

- Those individuals with significant pain may still benefit from intermittent short bouts of physical activity.

- Educate individuals to expect a small amount of discomfort in the muscles or joints during or after exercise is common. If individual's pain rating 2 hours after exercise is higher than it was prior to exercise, then the duration and/or intensity of future exercise sessions should be reduced.

Chapter 20—Electrocardiogram/Exercise for Rehabilitation   359

- Encourage individuals with arthritis to exercise during the time of day when pain is typically least severe and/or in conjunction with peak activity of pain medications.

- Appropriate shoes that provide shock absorption and stability are particularly important for individuals with arthritis. Shoe specialists can provide recommendations for appropriate shoes to meet individual biomechanical profiles.

- Incorporate functional exercises such as the sit-to-stand and step-ups as tolerated to improve neuromotor control, balance, and maintenance of activities of daily living (ADL)

- For water exercise, the temperature should be 83° to 88° F because warm water helps to relax muscles and reduce pain.

CANCER

The lifetime prevalence of cancer is roughly one in two for men and one in three for women. Cancer is most common in older individuals (≥55 years) and as a result there is increased likelihood that those with cancer will also have other chronic diseases (cardiovascular, pulmonary, diabetes, osteoporosis, and arthritis).

Exercise Testing and Cancer

Understanding how an individual has been affected by cancer is important prior to exercise testing and developing an exercise prescription. Must take into consideration cancer site-specific recommendations of the medical assessment.

Standard GXT procedures are generally appropriate with the following special considerations:

- Ideally, cancer survivors should have a comprehensive assessment of all health related components of physical fitness unless they pose as a barrier to initiation of a physical activity program.

- Be aware of co-morbid chronic diseases and other health conditions.

Exercise Prescription and Cancer

Frequency: For those who have completed treatment, the goal is 3 to 5 days per week with resistance training 2 to 3 days per week. Those currently undergoing treatment can increase daily physical activity sessions over the course of 1 month.

Intensity: If tolerated without adverse effects of symptoms or side effects, exercise intensity need not differ from healthy populations. However, exercise tolerance can be highly variable during active treatment and must be adjusted accordingly.

Time: During active treatment, multiple short bouts throughout the day may be beneficial. For survivors of cancer, time of physical activity guidelines should follow those of healthy individuals.

Type: Aerobic exercise should be prolonged, rhythmic activities using large muscle groups. Resistance exercise should be weights, resistance machines, etc targeting all major muscle groups. Flexibility and range of motion exercises should address specific areas of joint or muscle restriction that may have resulted from cancer-related treatment.

Progression: Progression may be slower in cancer survivors compared to healthy controls.

Special Considerations for Cancer

- Up to 90% of cancer survivors will experience cancer-related fatigue.

- Bone is a common site of metastases for many types of cancer. Modify the exercise prescription to reduce impact, intensity, and volume in those types of cancers with high risk of bone metastasis.

OSTEOPOROSIS

A condition characterized by low bone mineral density that increases susceptibility to fracture. More than 10 million people in the United States have osteoporosis with an additional 34 million at risk. Defined in postmenopausal women and in men ≥50 years old as a BMD T-score of lumbar spine, total hip, or femoral neck of ≤ –2.5. Physical activity plays a vital role in the primary and secondary prevention of osteoporosis.

Exercise Testing and Osteoporosis

The following issues should be considered when performing exercise testing in those individuals with osteoporosis:

- Cycle ergometry testing may be beneficial in those with severe vertebral osteoporosis.
- Vertebral compression fractures causing spinal deformation can result in reduced ventilatory capacity and a forward shift in the center of gravity (balance issues).
- Although there are no established guidelines for maximal muscle strength testing in individuals with osteoporosis, one repetition maximum testing may be contraindicated in those with severe osteoporosis.

Exercise Prescription and Individuals at Risk for Osteoporosis

Frequency: Weight bearing aerobic activities 3 to 5 days per week and resistance exercises 2 to 3 days per week.

Intensity: Moderate to vigorous intensity aerobic exercise. Moderate to vigorous resistance exercise.

Time: 30 to 60 minutes per day of a combination of weight-bearing aerobic and resistance activities.

Type: Weight-bearing aerobic and resistance exercise.

Exercise Prescription and Individuals with Osteoporosis

Frequency: Weight-bearing aerobic activities 3 to 5 days per week and resistance exercise 2 to 3 days per week.

Intensity: Moderate weight-bearing aerobic and resistance activities.

Time: 30 to 60 minutes per day of a combination of weight-bearing aerobic and resistance activities.

Type: Weight-bearing aerobic and resistance exercise.

PULMONARY DISEASE

Patients with pulmonary disease who benefit from physical activity include:

- COPD

  Bronchitis

Emphysema

- Asthma: Airway obstruction due to inflammation and bronchospasm
- Cystic fibrosis: Genetic disease resulting in excessive, thick mucus that obstructs the airways.
- Bronchiectasis: Chronic enlargement of the airways with impaired mucus clearance.
- Pulmonary fibrosis: Scarring and thickening of the parenchyma of the lungs.
- Lung cancer: Cigarette smoking

Asthma and Exercise Testing

- Functional capacity should be determined through CPET, pulmonary function testing, and oxyhemoglobin saturation.
- Administration of inhaled bronchodilator prior to CPET may be used to prevent exercise induced bronchoconstriction.

Exercise Prescription and Asthma

Frequency: At least 2 to 3 days per week

Intensity: At ventilatory threshold or at least 60% Vo_2 peak or 80% of maximal walking speed from 6-minute walk.

Chapter 20—Electrocardiogram/Exercise for Rehabilitation   363

Time: At least 20 to 30 minutes per day

Type: Aerobic activities using large muscle groups. Swimming in nonchlorinated pool is less asthmogenic.

Progression: As tolerated, progress to approximately 70% VO_2 peak.

Special Considerations and Asthma

- Should not exercise if experiencing acute asthma attack.

Exercise Testing and COPD

- Assessment should include VO_2max, pulmonary function, and arterial oxygen saturation.

- Dyspnea should be quantified using validated scales.

- Duration of GXT should be between 5 and 9 minutes in those with severe COPD.

Exercise Prescription and COPD

Frequency: Minimum 3 to 5 days per week

Intensity: Vigorous (60 to 80% peak work rates) and light (30 to 40% peak work rates) intensity.

Light intensity training results in improvements in symptoms, health-related quality of life, and performance of ADL. Vigorous intensity has been shown to result in greater physiologic improvements (e.g., reduced minute ventilation and HR at a given workload). Intensity may be based on a dyspnea rating of between 4 and 6 on the Borg CR10 Scale.

Time: Possible interval training

Type: Walking and/or cycling.

Special Considerations and COPD

- COPD and other pulmonary diseases affect not only the lungs, but also skeletal muscle. Resistance training should be encouraged.

- To help reduce dyspnea with normal activities of daily living, encourage resistance exercises of the shoulder girdle.

- Inspiratory muscle training is recommended for those with COPD and inspiratory muscle weakness.

- Consider prescribing exercise intensities using dyspnea scales.

Unlike most healthy individuals and individuals with CVD, patients with moderate-to-severe COPD may exhibit oxyhemoglobin desaturation with exercise. Therefore, a measure of blood oxygenation, either the partial pressure of arterial oxygen (PaO2) or %SaO2, should be made during the initial GXT. In addition, oximetry is recommended for the initial exercise training sessions to evaluate possible exercise-induced oxyhemoglobin desaturation and to identify the workload at which desaturation occurred.

Supplemental oxygen (O2) is indicated for patients with a PaO2 ≤55 mm Hg or a %SaO2 ≤88% while breathing room air. These same guidelines apply when considering supplemental oxygen during exercise.

In selected patients with severe COPD, using noninvasive positive pressure ventilation as an adjunct to exercise training produces modest gains in exercise performance. Because of the difficulty administering such an intervention, it is only recommended in those patients with advanced disease.

Individuals suffering from acute exacerbations of their pulmonary disease should limit exercise until symptoms have subsided.

Review Questions for Chapter 20

(For true and false questions that are false, indicate what would make the statement true)

1. Discuss the three bipolar limb leads in terms of the names of the leads and the anatomical locations on the body of the electrodes that make up these leads.

2. The paired leads of the heart that are said to be specific to the inferior portion of the heart are:

   a. Leads I and aVL

   b. Leads II, III, and aVF

   c. Leads V1, V2, V3 and V4

   d. Leads V5 and V6

3. The paired leads of the heart that are said to be specific to the high lateral portion of the heart are:

   a. Leads I and aVL

   b. Leads II, III, and aVF

   c. Leads V1, V2, V3 and V4

   d. Leads V5 and V6

4. The paired leads of the heart that are said to be specific to the anterior / septal wall of the heart are:

   a. Leads I and aVL

   b. Leads II, III, and aVF

   c. Leads V1, V2, V3 and V4

   d. Leads V5 and V6

5. A normal PR interval is defined as:

   a. < 120 ms

   b. < .12 sec

   c. 0.12 sec – 0.20 sec

   d. > 0.20 sec

6. Describe the three different AV blocks associated with a prolonged PR interval.

7. A normal QRS duration is defined as:

   a. < 120 ms

   b. < .12 sec

   c. 0.12 sec – 0.20 sec

   d. > 0.20 sec

Chapter 20—Electrocardiogram/Exercise for Rehabilitation   367

8. Describe the different types of blocks associated with prolonged QRS duration

9. Explain the difference between myocardial ischemia and myocardial infarction. Be sure to include in your discussion how these conditions may present on an ECG.

10. The severity of coronary artery disease and resulting ischemia during CPET is often said to be:

    a. Proportional to the magnitude of ST segment depression on ECG

    b. Proportional to the number of leads showing ST segment abnormalities on the ECG

    c. Proportional to the duration of ST segment depression into recovery

    d. A and B are correct

    e. A, B and C are correct

11. Discuss the impact of positive or negative ST-segment responses during a CPET on the posttest probability of angiographically significant CVD in subjects with different pretest probabilities (e.g., someone who is low risk vs moderate risk vs high risk for cardiovascular disease).

12. True / False: The motorized treadmill is the most often used type of exercise during a Cardiopulmonary exercise test.

13. True / False: Individuals are more likely to reach their true maximal effort when exercising on a cycle ergometer.

14. Which of the following conditions is considered to be an absolute indication for terminating an exercise test?

    a. Drop in systolic BP of $\geq$ 10 mmHg with an increase in work rate without the presence of other evidence of ischemia.

    b. Subject request to stop

    c. ST depression of 1 mm that is horizontal

    d. Fatigue and shortness of breath

15. Discuss the difference between absolute vs relative indications for stopping a CPET. How do these conditions affect the CPET?

16. The minimum standard criteria for a positive test of possible ischemia in terms of ECG response is what?

   a. ≥ 1.0 mm of upsloping ST segment depression

   b. ≥ 1.0 mm of horizontal or downsloping ST segment depression

   c. ≥ 2.0 mm of ST segment depression

17. The slope of the ST segment is typically measured starting at the J point extending for what duration?

   a. 20 ms

   b. 40 ms

   c. 60 – 80 ms

   d. 100 ms

18. True / False: The presence and duration of ST segment abnormalities during recovery provide little evidence to the presence of cardiovascular disease.

19. In terms of ischemic severity, the most severe ischemia is most often seen as:

   a. Upsloping ST segment depression

   b. Horizontal ST segment depression

   c. Upsloping ST segment depression

20. True / False: The reduction or suppression of ventricular arrhythmias (e.g., PVC) with physical activity usually indicates the absence of CVD.

21. The normal heart rate response to increasing exercise intensity is reported to be approximately?

   a. Increase of 5 bpm / 1 MET level of activity

   b. Increase of 10 bpm / 1 MET level of activity

   c. Increase of 20 bpm / 1 MET level of activity

   d. Increase of 30 bpm / 1 MET level of activity

22. Explain what chronotropic incompetence is and how it is measured.

23. Which CPET variable is sometimes referred to as the "Poor man's measure of stroke volume"?

   a. VO_2 – Work rate relationship

   b. O_2 Pulse

   c. Ventilatory Reserve

   d. Heart rate reserve

24. In healthy individuals, the heart rate reserve at peak exercise should be approximately what?

   a. Less than 30 bpm

   b. Less than 20 bpm

   c. Less than 15 bpm

25. A person who has a small ventilatory reserve and a large heart rate reserve at peak exercise is likely dealing with what type of disease?

   a. Cardiovascular

   b. Pulmonary

   c. Metabolic

26. Which of the following are goals for inpatient Rehabilitation?

   a. Offset effects of bed rest

   b. Provide additional medical surveillance

   c. Identify patients with impairments influencing prognosis

   d. All of the above

27. Describe the exercise prescription for an inpatient cardiac rehabilitation patient utilizing the FITT principle.

28. _____ is a chronic systemic inflammatory disease in which there is pathological activity of the immune system against joint tissue.

   a. COPD

   b. Osteoarthritis

   c. Rheumatoid arthritis

   d. Osteoporosis

29. _____ is a condition characterized by low bone mineral density.

   a. COPD

   b. Osteoarthritis

   c. Rheumatoid arthritis

   d. Osteoporosis

30. True / False: Maximal muscle strength testing is always contraindicated in individuals with Osteoporosis due to the increased risk of bone fracture.

31. In COPD patients the HR-VO$_2$ slope is usually
    a. The same as in healthy individuals
    b. Steeper than compared to healthy individuals
    c. Less than compared to healthy individuals

32. True / False: Because osteoarthritis is a degenerative disease affecting the joints, these individuals should never engage in high intensity exercise or resistance training.

33. Which of the following statements are correct for individuals with arthritis?
    a. Individuals who are experiencing an acute flare up of arthritis should never perform physical activity until the flare up is resolved.
    b. Since these individuals will be training at low to moderate intensity, they do not need to perform a warm up or cool down.
    c. If an individual's pain rating 2 hours after exercise is higher than it was prior to exercise, then the duration and/or intensity of future exercise sessions should be reduced
    d. Both A and C are correct
    e. A, B, and C are all correct

34. For individuals who are at risk for developing bone cancer, how should the exercise prescription be modified?
    a. Remove all resistance training
    b. Reduce exercise intensity
    c. Physical activity should be avoided in this population

35. Which type of physical activity would be the most beneficial for individuals with osteoporosis?
    a. Walking
    b. Stationary cycling
    c. Swimming

36. The heart is a muscle and is susceptible to hypertrophy if forced to work against a resistance. Knowing the flow of blood through the heart, which chamber of the heart would likely become enlarged and change the force vector (and axis) if the patient had **pulmonary hypertension** ?

37. The two (2) most common types of arthritis are _____ and _____ arthritis.

Chapter 20—Electrocardiogram/Exercise for Rehabilitation   371

38. The greatest risk to exercising an individual with Osteoporosis is the risk of causing a bone _____ of the vertebra or the neck of the femur.

39. The most common side-effect of many cancer-related treatments is _____.

40. In the treatment of the pulmonary patient, two conditions are generally monitored and are the biggest concern during exercise. Shortness of breath is typically referred to as _____, while a lack of oxygen is termed _____.

SECTION TWO: LABORATORY ASSIGNMENTS

Unit One Laboratories

Name: _____

Endocrine Physiology Lab

INTRODUCTION

The endocrine portion of the pancreas functions primarily in the regulation of glucose homeostasis. The cells in the endocrine portion of the pancreas are located in the Islets of Langerhans, so named as they form islands of endocrine cells in a sea of exocrine glands. The beta and alpha cells located in the Islets produce the counterregulatory hormones, insulin and glucagon, respectively. The primary function of insulin is to lower blood glucose whereas glucagon acts to increase blood glucose levels. Together these hormones help maintain glucose homeostasis in the body.

CAUTION: Procedures in this exercise involve the use of human blood which puts you at risk of contamination and development of certain life-threatening communicable diseases including, but not limited to, AIDS and Hepatitis.

NOTE: This lab is not intended to provide diagnoses of any kind. The results are for instructional use only. If you are concerned about any results you may find, please consult your physician.

OBJECTIVES

To measure blood glucose (sugar) levels.

To gain an understanding of pancreatic function and homeostatic mechanisms in the endocrine system.

Performance of a Finger Stick

- The best locations for finger sticks are the third and fourth fingers of the nondominant hand. Do not use the tip of the finger or the center of the finger.

- Avoid the side of the finger where there is less soft tissue.

- Avoid the using the second (index) finger.

- Avoid puncturing a finger that is cold or cyanotic, swollen, scarred, or covered with a rash.

- Using a sterile lancet, make a skin puncture just off the center of the finger pad.

- Collect drops of blood into the collection device by gently massaging the finger.

- Follow the below instructions to mix the blood that is collected.

Unit One Laboratories   373

GLUCOSE TOLERANCE TEST PROTOCOL

Initial Blood Draw

- Sit down prior to pricking your finger.

- Clean the area to be pricked with an alcohol pad and dry completely.

- Prick the fingertip with a lancet.

- Hold the finger until a small drop of blood appears. You may need to apply a little pressure by squeezing the fingertip. Collect the blood drop with the test strip.

- Follow the instructions for inserting the test strip and using the meter.

- **IMPORTANT: Be sure to write down this value on your worksheet.**

- Dispose of lancets in the red biohazard sharps container.

Testing Procedure

- After the initial blood draw, drink the provided sports beverage. Be sure to drink it as quickly as possible.

- Repeat the blood draw and glucose testing everyone 30 minutes following the glucose drink for a total of two more tests over the course of 60 minutes.

- **IMPORTANT: Be sure to write down these values on your worksheet.**

Low-Intensity Exercise

Initial Blood Draw

- Sit down prior to pricking your finger.

- Clean the area to be pricked with an alcohol pad and dry completely.

- Prick the fingertip with a lancet.

- Hold the finger until a small drop of blood appears. You may need to apply a little pressure by squeezing the fingertip. Collect the blood drop with the test strip.

- Follow the instructions for inserting the test strip and using the meter.

- **IMPORTANT: Be sure to write down this value on your worksheet.**

- Dispose of lancets in the red biohazard sharps container.

Testing Procedure

- After the initial blood draw, start the treadmill and walk at 3.0 mph for 30 minutes.

- Repeat the blood draw and glucose testing following the 30 minutes of exercise

- **IMPORTANT: Be sure to write down this value on your worksheet.**

High-Intensity Exercise

Initial Blood Draw

- Sit down prior to pricking your finger.

- Clean the area to be pricked with an alcohol pad and dry completely.

- Prick the fingertip with a lancet.

- Hold the finger until a small drop of blood appears. You may need to apply a little pressure by squeezing the fingertip. Collect the blood drop with the test strip.

- Follow the instructions for inserting the test strip and using the meter.

- **IMPORTANT: Be sure to write down this value on your worksheet.**

- Dispose of lancets in the red biohazard sharps container.

Testing Procedure

- After the initial blood draw, start the treadmill and run at a comfortable pace for 15 minutes. After the 15-minute run complete a 30-second Wingate test.

- Repeat the blood draw and glucose testing following the Wingate test.

- **IMPORTANT: Be sure to write down this value on your worksheet.**

Unit One Laboratories   375

Worksheet: Results of Glucose Testing

Name: _____

GLUCOSE TOLERANCE TEST

Initial glucose reading (mg/dL): _____

Glucose at 30 mins (mg/dL): _____

Glucose at 60 mins (mg/dL): _____

Has the subject had any caffeine prior to this test? YES NO

If so, at what time? _____

What type of caffeine? _____

Did the subject have anything to eat prior to this lab? YES NO

If yes, at what time was your last meal? _____

LOW-INTENSITY EXERCISE

Initial glucose reading (mg/dL): _____

Glucose after 30 mins of low intensity exercise (mg/dL): _____

Has the subject had any caffeine prior to this test? YES NO

If so, at what time? _____

What type of caffeine? _____

Did the subject have anything to eat prior to this lab? YES NO

If yes, at what time was your last meal? _____

HIGH-INTENSITY EXERCISE

Initial glucose reading (mg/dL):_____

Glucose after 30 mins of high intensity exercise
(mg/dl):_____

Has the subject had any caffeine prior to this test? YES NO

If so, at what time? _____

What type of caffeine? _____

Did the subject have anything to eat prior to this lab? YES NO

If yes, at *what* time was your last meal? _____

Unit One Laboratories   377

Endocrine Questions:

1.   a.   What would you expect to happen to the blood glucose values over time after consuming a carbohydrate source?

      b.   Why would you expect the blood glucose to change?

2.   Describe what kind of changes in blood glucose you would expect to see from each of the following individuals:

      a.   Individual with peripheral insulin resistance

      b.   Aerobically-trained individual

3.   a.   What would you expect to happen to the blood glucose values after exercising for 60 minutes at 60% VO_2max? Following exercise of 120% VO_2max?

      b.   Explain why there may be a difference (be sure to include the endocrine mechanism)

Immune Lab Procedure

Name: _____

LABORATORY PROCEDURES

1. Two students will serve as the subject.

2. One subject will perform a VO_2max test and the other subject will work out for 30 minutes at 60% of their VO_2max.

    a. 60% of Vo_2max corresponds with 75% of maximum heart rate.

3. Each subject will perform a finger stick before and after the exercise testing, to determine their WBC.

4. Measure HR and RPE at every minute for each of the subjects.

Performance of a Finger Stick

-   The best locations for finger sticks are the third and fourth fingers of the nondominant hand. Do not use the tip of the finger or the center of the finger.

-   Avoid the side of the finger where there is less soft tissue.

-   Avoid the using the second (index) finger.

-   Avoid puncturing a finger that is cold or cyanotic, swollen, scarred, or covered with a rash.

-   Using a sterile lancet, make a skin puncture just off the center of the finger pad.

-   Collect drops of blood into the collection device by gently massaging the finger.

-   Follow the below instructions to mix the blood that is collected.

Unit One Laboratories   379

WBC Determination

HEMACYTOMETER

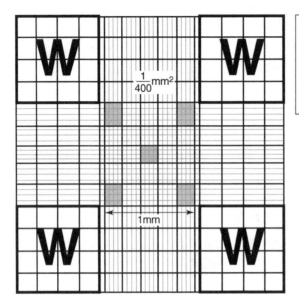

The four corner primary squares are used when counting leukocytes. These four large corner squares contain 16 smaller secondary squares.

LEUKOCHEK TEST KIT

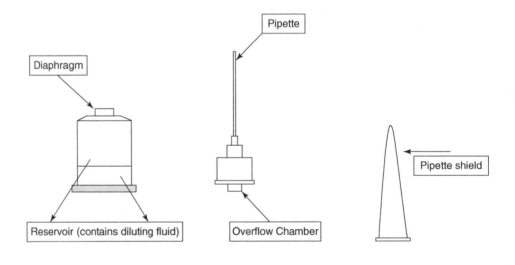

Procedure for Counting WBCs

a. Leukocytes are counted in the FOUR OUTSIDE LARGE squares of the counting chamber.

b. Count the cells starting in the upper left top large corner square. Move to the upper right corner square, bottom right corner square, and end in the bottom left corner square.

c. Count all cells that touch any of the upper and left lines; do not count any cell that touches a lower or right line.

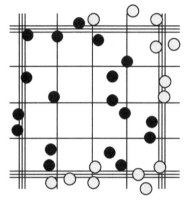

d. Calculation for counting four large squares:

  i. Use the number of cells counted in the hemocytometer.

  ii. Final cell count is reported as the number of white blood cells per microliter (WBC/μL).

  iii. Formula:

  $$\text{WBC}/\mu L = \frac{\text{Number of cells counted} \times \text{Correction for dilution}}{\text{Number of squares counted} \times \text{Volume of one square}}$$

  Correction for dilution = dilution factor, 1/100, so the dilution factor is 100

  Number of squares counted = four (4)

  Volume of one large square = 0.1 μL

  Example:

  Number of cells counted = 28

  $$\text{WBC}/\mu L = \frac{28 \times 100}{4 \times 0.1} = 7.0 \times 10^3/\mu L$$

EXPECTED NORMAL VALUES

Age	Range (10³/μL)
Newborn	9.0–30.0
1 week	5.0–21.0
1 month	5.0–19.5
6–12 months	6.0–17.5
2 years	6.2–17.0
Child/Adult	4.8–10.8

Test Sheet:

Name: _____

TRIAL: 60% OF VO$_{2MAX}$

Subject Name: _____ HR Max: _____

75% HR Max _____

Pretest WBC/μL: _____ Posttest WBC/μL: _____

Calculations for results:

TRIAL: VO$_{2MAX}$ TEST

Subject Name: _____ HR Max: _____

Pretest WBC/μL: _____ Posttest WBC/μL: _____

Calculations for results:

Test Sheet:

Name: _____

VO$_{2max}$ subject: _____   75% of VO$_{2max}$ subject: _____

Time	HR (bpm)	RPE	HR (bpm)	RPE
0				
1				
2				
3				
4				
5				
6				
7				
8				
9				
10				
11				
12				
13				
14				
15				
16				
17				
18				
19				
20				
21				
22				
23				
24				
25				
26				
27				
28				
29				
30				

Unit One Laboratories   385

Immune Questions:

1. Acute exercise can cause significant changes to the immune system during the ***actual exercise session.***

   a. Define and explain the process of **leukocytosis**.

   b. How might exercising to maximum affect this process differently than exercising for 30 minutes at 60% VO_2max?

   c. Did the results of your lab turn out the way you expected? Why or Why not?

2. Acute exercise can also affect the immune system ***post exercise.***

   a. Briefly discuss how high-intensity, long-duration exercise would affect the post-exercise immune response differently than moderate-intensity, short-duration exercise.

   b. Indicate how these two situations would affect:

      i. Lymphocyte number and function (give specific examples)

      ii. NK cell number and function

      iii. IgA function

3. Indicate how the ***endocrine system*** could affect the immune response to:

   a. A maximal bout of exercise (give specific examples)

386   Unit One Laboratories

b. Exercising for 30 minutes at 60% Vo_2max (give specific examples)

4. Define and briefly describe the **open window hypothesis.**

5. Briefly discuss how the two exercise sessions done in lab could affect the **general health** of an individual if done **chronically** (5 to 7 days each week over several months)

Unit Two Laboratories

Name: _____

Body Composition Assessment

INTRODUCTION

The purpose of this laboratory is to introduce and demonstrate various techniques of body composition analysis. The laboratory will focus on the principles and methodology of skinfold assessment of body composition, but will also introduce other means to analyze body composition, BMI, and waist-to-hip ratio (WHR).

Body composition is a term referring to the components of the human body. In this lab we will talk about two main components, fat free mass (FFM) and fat mass.

METHODS TO DETERMINE BODY COMPOSITION VIA SKINFOLD MEASURES

Because of the inherent error in estimating body composition via the skinfold measurements, it is crucial to utilize proper procedures when performing skin-fold analysis.

Subject Position

All skinfold sites are measured with the subject standing, and all sites are taken on the same side of the body.

Skinfold Technique

While holding the caliper with the right hand, the technician uses the thumb and index finger of the left hand to pinch the skinfold at a distance of about 1 cm proximal (towards the trunk of the body) to the skinfold site (or mark). This fold represents two layers of skin and fat (not the muscle). The long axis of the fold is a natural one, which is smooth and untwisted. This may be referred to as the natural cleavage of the skin. The caliper should be placed across the long axis (natural angle) of the skinfold. The jaws of the caliper should not press longer than 2 to 4 seconds at the skinfold site so they do not force fluid from the tissues and reduce the measurement. While still holding the skinfold with the thumb and index finger, the technician reads the gauge of the skinfold caliper to the nearest 2 mm mark.

Unit Two Laboratories   389

Number of Measurements

Three measurements at each skinfold site should be used during skinfold assessment. The technician should make a complete circuit of the measurement sites on the same side of the body, then repeat the circuit. This means that one of the skinfold should be measured and not repeated until all other skinfold sites are measured. The mean value of the three trials is used for evaluation.

Equations to Determine Body Density and Percent Body Fat

The equations used in most instances were developed by Jackson and Pollock. These equations typically use 7, 4, or 3 sites and various skinfold sites to measure either body density or percent body fat. Typically, the equations used will determine body density and will require and additional equation to determine percent body fat.

If an equation is used that calculated body density, a second equation is needed to convert body density to percent body fat. The most commonly used equation is Siri. The equation is listed below:

$$\textbf{\% Body fat = (495 / body density)} - \textbf{450} \quad \textbf{(Siri)}$$

Equations to Determine Amount of Fat and Lean Mass

- **Calculate fat weight**
  - FW (kg) = BW (kg) × % BF
    - % BF is in decimal form (13% = 0.13)
- **Calculate fat-free weight (Lean body weight)**

  FFW (kg) = BW (kg) × (1 − % BF)
- **Calculate Ideal Body Weight**

  IBW (kg) = FFW / (1 − desired % BF)

OTHER ANTHROPOMETRIC MEASUREMENTS

BMI

BMI is derived from body mass and stature and is frequently used by clinicians and researchers to evaluate the normalcy of one's body weight. BMI is calculated using the following equation:

$$\text{BMI} = \text{body mass, kg} / \text{height, m}^2$$

The importance of this easy-to-obtain index lies in its curvilinear relationship to the all-cause mortality ratio: as the BMI becomes larger, so also does the risk of a variety of diseases, such as cardiovascular complications, diabetes, and renal disease. Norm charts and tables for BMI are provided on SOLE.

390   Unit Two Laboratories

Waist-to-Hip Ratio

Waist is the smallest circumference. Usually above the umbilicus. Hip is the widest part of the hips and buttocks

Waist circumference (cm)/hip circumference (cm)

LABORATORY PROCEDURES

1. Students will get into groups of two individuals and practice taking skinfold measurements at 3 sites and 7 sites.

2. Each technician's measurements will be recorded on the subject's data sheet. Make sure to use the proper protocols as outlined in the laboratory.

3. Each subject will then complete BMI and WHR. Record **your own** data on the data sheet.

DATA SHEET

Name (M): _____ Age: _____ Body weight (kg): _____

Name (F): _____ Age: _____ Body weight (kg): _____

7-site skinfold

Male	Trial 1	Trial 2	Trial 3	Ave.
Chest				
Abdomen				
Thigh				
Tricep				
Suprailiac				
Midaxillary				
Subscapular				

Female	Trial 1	Trial 2	Trial 3	Ave.
Chest				
Abdomen				
Thigh				
Tricep				
Suprailiac				
Midaxillary				
Subscapular				

3-site skinfold, female

Site	Trial 1	Trial 2	Trial 3	Ave.
Triceps				
Suprailiac				
Thigh				

3-site skinfold, male

Site	Trial 1	Trial 2	Trial 3	Ave.
Chest				
Abdomen				
Thigh				

BMI

Body weight (kg): _____ Height: _____ cm _____ m^2

BMI: _____

Show calculations:

Waist- to- Hip Ratio

Waist circumference: _____cm Hip circumference: _____ cm

Waist- to- Hip Ratio:_____

Show calculations:

Questions

1. Calculate percent body fat of your 7- and 3-site data. Utilize the Brozek equation (in lab) to convert body density to percent body fat when necessary. Show all calculations and organize and label your calculations so the information can be easily read.

2. Utilizing the percent body fat from the 7-site equation, calculate fat weight and fat-free weight from each technician's values. Also, calculate ideal body weight (assume an ideal % body fat of 15% for males and 22% for females) using the fat-free weight value from the 7-site equation.

3. Compare your waist- to- hipratio, BMI, and 3-site skinfold tests and determine where you fall in terms of health risks for each. Do all three agree on the same conclusion? If not, explain why there may be contradictions?

4. Explain some factors that may contribute to measurement error within skinfold assessment?

5. Explain and describe another method that would be more accurate in determining body composition.

Name: _____

Resting Metabolic Rate Laboratory

INTRODUCTION

Metabolic processes in the body require energy. The rate at which these processes occur is measured in calories per unit of time and is most often given in calories per day.

Basal metabolic rate (BMR): Each person requires a minimum level of energy to sustain vital functions in the waking state, this energy requirement is BMR. BMR can only be found during an awake but totally rested and postabsorptive state and in a neutrally temperate environment.

Resting metabolic rate (RMR): is the sum of metabolic processes of the active cell mass required to maintain normal regulatory balance and body functions at rest. RMR can be measured 3 to 4 hours after a light meal and no prior physical activity.

The total amount of calories an individual burns in a given day is known as total daily energy expenditure (TDEE).

TDEE = RMR + TEF + NEAT + EPOC + EX

- **TDEE** = total daily energy expenditure
- **RMR** = resting metabolic rate
- **TEF** = thermogenic effect of food
- **NEAT** = non-exercise activity thermogenesis
- **EPOC** = excess post-exercise oxygen consumption
- **EX** = exercise

RMR and TEF are constant, with minor fluctuations due to muscle mass, conditioning, and dietary shifts. NEAT and exercise have large variability and can greatly influence a person's total caloric expenditure.

Calculating RMR: The Weir equation (REE) can be used to calculate the number of calories burned per minute.

REE (resting energy expenditure) = $((3.9 (VO_2) + 1.1 (VCO_2)) \times 1.44$

- **Vo_2 = volume of oxygen uptake (mL/min)**
- **Vco_2 = volume of carbon dioxide output (mL/min)**

RMR can also be calculated using estimation formulas:

Revised Harris–Benedict BMR Equations (calories/day)

Male: $(88.4 + 13.4 \times weight) + (4.8 \times height) - (5.68 \times age)$

Female: $(447.6 + 9.25 \times weight) + (3.10 \times height) - (4.33 \times age)$

** weight in kilograms, height in centimeters, age in years

Unit Two Laboratories   397

Mifflin–St Jeor Equations (calories/day)

Male: (9.99 × weight) + (6.25 × height) − (4.92 × age) + 5

Female: (9.99 × weight) + (6.25 × height) − (4.92 × age) − 161

**weight in kilograms, height in centimeters, age in years

LABORATORY PROCEDURES

We are going to assess RMR in two different individuals at two different resting states.

Participant 1: will come to lab 12 hours fasted and 24 hours without physical activity/exercise

Participant 2: will come to lab after eating a meal and having an intense work out either the night before or the morning of lab

When the participants arrive in lab they will lay down and rest for 30 minutes after the 30 minutes we will obtain their VO_2 using the metabolic cart.

Participant	Activity Level	Height	Weight	Age	VO_2	VCO_2

Data for Participant 1 (show all work):

- **Weir Equation:**

  - **REE =**

- **Revised Harris–Benedict BMR Equations (calories/day)**

- **Mifflin–St Jeor Equations (calories/day)**

Data for Participant 2 (show all work):

- **Weir Equation:**
  - **REE =**

- **Revised Harris–Benedict BMR Equations (calories/day)**

- **Mifflin–St Jeor Equations (calories/day)**

Questions

1. When using the Harris–Benedict equation and the Mifflin–St. Jeor Equation, the calculation for calories used per day can be off as much as 1,000 calories. Why? And where does the majority of variation or error come from?

2. Show the results for the three above equations for each participant. Are there any differences between the three results? Why or Why not?

3. Can a person's resting metabolism be improved? Explain.

4. Explain why on average a person's resting metabolic rate declines as they age.

Assessing Physical Activity and Energy Expenditure

Name: _____

INTRODUCTION

The rates of individuals that are overweight or obese in the United States a has increased dramatically over the last 50 years and continue to rise. This weight gain in individuals is ultimately related to caloric balance:

Caloric balance = the amount of energy consumed − the amount of energy expended

The reason that obesity rates have increased is because there is an increase in consumption of food and a decrease in energy expended.

Energy is expended in three ways: resting metabolic rate (approximately 67%), physical activity and NEAT (approximately 23%), and the thermogenic effect of food (approximately 10%). The percentages listed are averages and can vary greatly depending on the amount of physical activity an individual participates in.

Physical activity is any form of movement. Physical activity may include planned activity/exercise (running) as well as any other daily activities (yard work).

Physical activity can be quantified in a variety of ways. Some examples:

- **Indirect calorimetry**—The estimation of energy expenditure via the measurement of oxygen consumption and carbon dioxide production.

- **Accelerometer**—An instrument that measures acceleration. The measures of acceleration are then converted into a mathematical unit. Those units (in some accelerometers) have been deemed by multiple scientists to be valid estimates of physical activity. In certain models those units can be converted into METs or calories expended, therefore accelerometers can estimate the intensity of an activity.

- **Pedometer**—A device that counts the number of strides taken by the wearer by responding to the impact of the wearer's steps. The pedometer responds to the percussive movements of feet hitting the ground and provides only a count of the number of steps taken. It does not provide a measure of intensity.

- **Self-report**—Person in question reports when they were active, the type, and duration of activity.

Unit Two Laboratories   403

LABORATORY PROCEDURES

We are going to use one method to assess different types of activity.

Method 1: Indirect calorimetry

This method will be utilized to collect data during the following six activities:

1. Resting with no weight: Participant will rest in a recumbent position for 15 minutes.

2. Resting with weight (25 pounds): Participant will rest in a recumbent position with weight for 15 minutes.

3. Treadmill with no weight: Participant will walk at comfortable pace on the treadmill for 15 minutes.

4. Treadmill with weight (25 pounds): Participant will walk at same pace on the treadmill with weight added on for 15 minutes.

5. Bike with no weight: Participant will bike at a comfortable pace for 15 minutes.

6. Bike with weight (25 pounds): Participant will bike at the same pace with weight added on for 15 minutes.

You will collect VO_2 data for each activity in class and enter that data in the table below:

Convert VO_2 $mL \cdot kg^{-1} \cdot min^{-1}$ into METs:

$$METs = VO_2 \, mL \cdot kg^{-1} \cdot min^{-1} / 3.5$$

Convert VO_2 L/min into kcals/min:

$$kcals/min = VO_2 \, L/min \times 5$$

Participant Name:

Age:

Body weight: Body weight after weight added on:

Activity	V_{O_2} mL·kg^{-1}·min^{-1}
Resting with no weight	
Resting with weight	

Participant Name:

Age:

Body weight: Body weight after weight added on:

Activity	V_{O_2} mL·kg^{-1}·min^{-1}
Treadmill with no weight	
Treadmill with weight	

Participant Name:

Age:

Body weight: Body weight after weight added on:

Activity	V_{O_2} mL·kg^{-1}·min^{-1}
Bike with no weight	
Bike with weight	

Unit Two Laboratories   405

Questions

1. Show all calculations of converting VO_2 data from rest, treadmill, and bike (with and without weight) into METs and kcal/min.

2. Would there be any discrepancies between the VO_2 data and accelerometer data (if used)? If so, why may these discrepancies occur?

3. What are some advantages and disadvantages of using a pedometer, accelerometer, or self- report?

4. Do heavier or lighter individuals expend more total energy? Why? What types of activities would expend the most energy?

Name: _____

Pediatric Fitness Assessment

INTRODUCTION

There is no denying that kids today are heavier than kids in the past. Nearly 1 in 5 children in the United States are obese. Many factors contribute to childhood obesity; genetics, metabolism, eating and physical activity behaviors. As a greater number of younger individuals, and their parents, seek personalized exercise programming, it is becoming essential in the clinical setting to have the knowledge and skills to accurately assess fitness levels in children.

Kids' fitness assessments provide a wealth of information. We can determine a child's strength and weaknesses. We can set realistic goals for a child and also educate the child about their fitness. Schools can use the data to design better physical activity programs. Overall, the end goal is to motivate children to embrace a active lifestyle and maintain it throughout adulthood.

Two of the most widely used testing programs for kids are the FITNESS program and the President's Challenge program.

AEROBIC CAPACITY TESTING

The PACER (Progressive Aerobic Cardiovascular Endurance Run)

The PACER is a multistage fitness test adapted from the 20-m shuttle run. The test is progressive in intensity; it is easy at the beginning and gets harder at the end.

The Objective: To run as long as possible with continuous movement back and forth across a 20-m space at a specified pace that gets faster each minute.

The One-Mile Run

The one-mile run can be used instead of the PACER to provide an estimate of aerobic capacity.

The Objective: To run a mile at the fastest pace possible. If a student cannot run the total distance, walking is permitted.

Scoring: The one-mile run is scored in minutes and seconds.

The Walk Test

Another alternative to the PACER is the one-mile walk test.

The Objective: To walk 1 mile as quickly as possible while maintaining a constant walking pace the entire distance.

Unit Two Laboratories   409

Scoring:

1. The walk test is scored in minutes and seconds.

2. A 60-second heart rate should be taken at the conclusion of the walk.

3. Estimated VO_2max is calculated using the RockPort Fitness Walking Test Equation:

VO_{2max} $(mL \cdot kg^{-1} \cdot min^{-1})$ = 132.853 − 0.1692 (body mass in kg) − 0.3877 (age in years) + 6.315 (gender) − 3.2649 (time in minutes) − 0.1565 (HR)

*(gender = 0 for female, 1 for male; HR is taken at end of walk)

BODY COMPOSITION

Skinfold Measurements

*See additional Handout from skinfold lab

Body Mass Index

The BMI provides an indication of the appropriateness of a child's weight relative to height. BMI is determined by the following formula:

$$weight \ (kg) \ / \ height^2 \ (m^2)$$

MUSCULAR STRENGTH, ENDURANCE AND FLEXIBILITY

The Curl-Up

The Objective: To complete as many curl-ups as possible up to a maximum of 75 at a specified pace.

Test Instructions:

1. Student lies in a supine position on the mat, knees bent at an angle of approximately 140 degrees, feet flat on the floor, legs slightly apart, arms straight and parallel to the trunk with palms of the hands resting on the mat.

2. The fingers are stretched out and the head is in contact with the mat.

3. Keeping heels in contact with the mat, student will slowly curl up to a halfway mark and then will curl back down until his or her head touches the mat.

4. Movement should be slow and gauged to the specified cadence of about 20 curl-ups per minute (1 curl up every 3 seconds).

Scoring:

1. The score is the number of curls-ups performed.

2. Curl-ups should be counted when the student's head returns to the mat.

410   Unit Two Laboratories

Trunk Lift

The Objective: To lift upper body off the floor using the muscles of the back and hold the position to allow for the measurement.

Test Instructions:

1. The student being tested lies on the mat in a prone position (facedown).

2. The toes are pointed and hands are placed under the thighs.

3. The student lifts the body off the floor in a very slow controlled manner to a maximum height of 12 inches.

4. The head should be maintained in a neutral alignment with the spine.

5. The position is held long enough to allow the tester to place the ruler on the floor in front of the student and determine the distance from the floor to the student's chin.

6. Once the measurement is made the student returns to the starting position. Allow two trials recording the highest score.

90° Push-up

The Objective: To complete as many 90° push-ups as possible at a rhythmic pace.

Test Instructions:

1. Student being tested assumes a prone position on the mat with hands placed under or slightly wider than the shoulders.

2. Fingers are stretched out, legs straight and slightly apart, and toes tucked under.

3. The student pushes up off the mat with the arms until the arms are straight, keeping the legs and back straight.

4. The back should be kept in a straight line from head to toes throughout the test.

5. The student then lowers the body using the arms until the elbow bend at a 90° angle and the upper arms are parallel to the floor.

6. This movement is repeated as many times as possible with no rest in between reps.

7. The student should push up and continue the movement until the arms are straight on each repetition.

8. The rhythm should be approximately 20 90° push-ups per minute or 1 90° push-up every 3 seconds.

Scoring: The number of push-ups performed.

Unit Two Laboratories   411

Back-Saver Sit and Reach

The Objective: To be able to reach the specified distance on both the right and left sides of the body.

Test Instructions:

1. Student should remove his or her shoes.

2. One leg is fully extended with the foot flat against the face of the box.

3. The other knee is bent with the sole of the foot flat on the floor.

4. The arms are extended forward over the measuring scale with the hands placed one on top of the other.

5. With palms down, the student reaches directly forward with both hands.

6. After one side has been measured, the student switches the position of the legs and reaches again.

Scoring: Record the number of inches on each side to the nearest ½ inch reached.

Shoulder Stretch

The Objective: To be able to touch the fingertips together behind the back by reaching over the shoulder and under the elbow.

Test Instructions:

1. To test the right shoulder, the student reaches with the right hand over the right shoulder and down the back.

2. At the same time, the student places the left hand behind the back and reaches up trying to touch the fingers of the right hand. The students' partner determines whether or not the fingers touch.

3. To test the left shoulder, the student reaches with the left hand over the left shoulder and down the back.

4. At the same, the student places the right hand behind the back and reaches up, trying to touch the fingers of the left hand. The students' partner determines whether or not the fingers touch.

Scoring:

1. If the student is able to touch his or her fingers with the left hand over the shoulder, a "Y" is recorded for the left side, if not an "N" is recorded.

2. If the student is able to touch his or her fingers with the right hand over the shoulder, a "Y" is recorded for the right side, if not an "N" is recorded.

SCORE SHEET

Participant's Name: _____

Height: _____   **Weight:** _____

BMI: _____

1-MW V_{O_2}	Curl-Up # completed	Trunk Lift Inches	Push-Up # completed	Sit and Reach Inches	Shoulder Stretch Right	Left

Questions for Pediatric Fitness Assessment:

1. How has childhood obesity changed in the past 50 years (increased or decreased) and why do you think that we have seen this change.

2. Why do we need youth fitness tests? Explain.

3. Explain the Kraus–Weber Minimal Fitness Test (one of the first children's fitness test).

4. What are some things to consider when testing a pediatric population? Explain.

Name: _____

Senior Fitness Test: Defining Functional Fitness Parameters

INTRODUCTION

A disability is one's inability to perform normal daily activities such as bathing oneself, housework, or shopping.

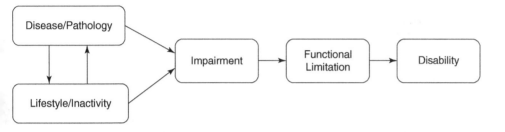

Physical impairments observed in the elderly are modifiable through assessment and activity intervention no matter the origin of the impairments.

There are several physical parameters that are essential components of functional fitness and include: muscular strength/endurance, aerobic endurance, flexibility, agility/dynamic balance, and BMI.

Muscular Strength

According to ACSM, muscular strength declines 15 to 20% per decade after the age of 50. Lack of muscular strength can hinder one's ability to perform several common tasks and is essential for fall related injury prevention.

Aerobic Endurance

It is estimated that a VO_2max if 15 to 18 mL/kg/min is required for one to maintain functional independence. Aerobic capacity declines at a rate of 5 to 15% per decade after the age of 30 but can be avoided through physical activity.

Flexibility

Loss of flexibility is associated with aging. According to ACSM, full range of motion of the hip and knee joint is essential for preventing falls, preventing back pain and musculoskeletal injuries, and maintaining proper gait patterns among older adults.

Agility/Dynamic Balance

Agility and dynamic balance are essential for numerous everyday tasks, Mos
importantly, agility and dynamic balance are essential for proper gait pattern
and fall prevention. Both agility and dynamic balance decline with age.

Body Mass Index

People with high BMI are more likely to become disabled; and people with low
BMI have mobility problems. On average, individuals gain 1 lb per year after
the age of 30 until the age of 50 or 60, after which time there is usually a slow
decline in weight.

Functional Fitness Tests

Assessment Category	Test Item	Description
Lower body strength	30-s chair stand	No. of full stands in 30s with arms folded across chest
upper body strength	Arm curl	No. of biceps curls in 30s holding hand weight (women 5 lb, men 8 lb)
Aerobic endurance	6-min walk 2-min step test (alternative aerobic test)	No. of yd walked in 6 min around a 50 yd course No. of full steps completed in 2 min, raising each knee to point midway between patella and iliac crest
Lower body flexibility	Chair sit-and-reach	From sitting position at front of chair, with leg extended and hands reaching toward toes, no. of inches (+ or −) from extended fingers to tip of toe
Upper body flexibility	Back scratch	With one hand reaching over shoulder and one up middle of back, no. of inches between extended middle fingers (+ or −)
Agility/Dynamic balance	8-foot up-and-go	No. of seconds required to rise from seated position, walk 8 ft, turn and return to a seated position on chair
Body composition	BMI	Ratio of body weight to height (kg/m^2)

DATA SHEET FOR FUNCTIONAL FITNESS ASSESSMENT

30s Chair stand	_____ no. of full stands
Arm curl	_____ no. of curls
2-min step test	_____ no. of full steps
Chair sit-and-reach	+ or –_____ inches
Back scratch	+ or –_____ inches
8-foot up-and-go	_____ no. of seconds
BMI	_____ (kg/m^2)

DATA SHEET FOR BERG BALANCE SCALE

Item Description	Score (0–4)
Sitting to standing	
Standing unsupported	
Sitting unsupported	
Standing to sitting	
Transfers	
Standing with eyes closed	
Standing with feet together	
Reaching forward with outstretched arm	
Retrieving object from floor	
Turning to look behind	
Turning 360 degrees	
Placing alternate foot on stool	
Standing with one foot in front	
Standing on one foot	

Total: _____

Risk Category: _____

Questions

1. What causes reduction in muscle strength between the ages of 25 and 80?

2. Biological aging relates to changes in three hormonal systems. What are they and explain each one.

3. Explain why an elderly individual should resistance train.

4. Explain how physical activity affects neural function, cardiovascular function, and body composition in older individuals.

Unit Three Laboratories

Name: _____

Cardiopulmonary Exercise Testing Laboratory (CPET): Hypoxic Exercise

Objective of this lab: To conduct a symptom-limited, submaximal cardiopulmonary exercise test at simulated altitude of approximately 6,000 ft (1800 m) and evaluate the ECG and open-circuit metabolic and ventilatory responses in healthy populations.

KEY CONCEPTS:

1. Ability to set up and prepare an individual for a CPET (hook up and administer 12-lead ECG, using metabolic systems such as the ParvoMedics to administer the appropriate CPET modality and device protocol).

2. Ability to generate summary and nine-panel reports following completion of a CPET.

3. Interpret and explain breath-by-breath changes at rest and during exercise for FeO_2, $FeCO_2$, VO_2, VCO_2, RER, Ve, Vt, RR, breathing reserve (BR), Ve/VO_2, Ve/VCO_2, HR, VO_2–workload relationship, HR–O_2 relationship, HRR, and O_2 pulse in healthy individuals exercising in hypoxia compared to normoxia.

INSTRUCTIONS

1. Have a subject (from the previous week's lab, for which data are available regarding a normoxia CPET), complete a physical activity readiness questionnaire (PAR-Q), and review the responses with your laboratory instructor.

2. Perform a modified 12-lead ECG hook-up so that the limb leads are moved from the distal limbs to the thorax.

    a. Be certain to practice the skills necessary during ECG hook-up to minimize ECG noise/artifact during exercise as well as to ensure participant safety while walking/cycling.

3. Calibrate the breath-by-breath metabolic system according to the manufacturer's instructions.

4. Set up the mouthpiece and head gear (including nose clips) of the metabolic system on the subject.

5. Enter the test subject's data into the metabolic system and choose maximal treadmill test as the type of test.

6. Select and perform the Bruce protocol in both the metabolic and ECG software.

Unit Three Laboratories   423

7. Record the rating of perceived exertion at the end of each stage.

8. Encourage the subject to continue to push until the subject requests to stop, fails to conform to the exercise protocol, develops adverse signs and/or symptoms, experiences any emergency situation, or reaches 75% of max HR (determined from normoxia CPET).

9. When the test is terminated, immediately begin the active recovery by clicking on the cool-down button, and allow the subject to continue walking at 0% elevation and 1.5 mph. At the same time, have a test technician immediately remove the mouthpiece and noseclips from the subject during the cool-down phase.

10. Upon completion of the test, print off a text report, summary report, and nine-panel report from the reports tab.

Questions

1. Record *resting* FeO_2, $FeCO_2$, VO_2, VCO_2, RER, Ve, Vt, RR, Ve/VO_2, Ve/VCO_2, and HR for this test and compare them to values previously obtained at rest (on the same person) in normoxia.

	Resting Normoxia Values	Resting Hypoxia Values
FeO_2		
$FeCO_2$		
VO_2		
VCO_2		
RER		
Ve		
Vt		
RR		
Ve/VO_2		
Ve/VCO_2		
HR		

Unit Three Laboratories   425

2. Record VO_2, VCO_2, RER, Ve, Vt, RR, Ve/VO_2, Ve/VCO_2, HR, the VO_2–workload relationship, the $HR-VO_2$ relationship at Stages I and III, and the highest stage achieved in during the hypoxia test; compare these to the same variables obtained at the same exercise stages in the normoxia CPET.

	Stage I		Stage III		Highest Stage	
	Normoxia	Hypoxia	Normoxia	Hypoxia	Normoxia	Hypoxia
FeO_2						
$FeCO_2$						
VO_2						
VCO_2						
RER						
Ve						
Vt						
RR						
Ve/VO_2						
Ve/VCO_2						
HR						
VO_2–workload relationship						
$HR-VO_2$ relationship						

426   Unit Three Laboratories

3. Plot ventilation obtained from rest and during exercise in normoxia and hypoxia (data from questions 1 and 2) on the following graph.

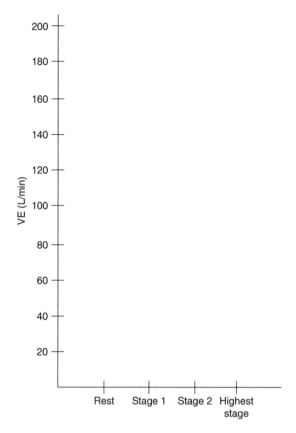

4. Plot heart rate obtained from rest and during exercise in normoxia and hypoxia (data from questions 1 and 2) on the following graph.

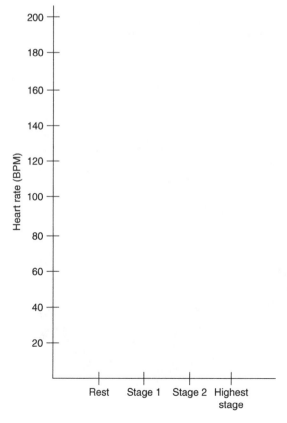

Unit Three Laboratories 427

5. Calculate the % difference of ventilation in hypoxia compared to normoxia for rest and each exercise level (using previously obtained data) and provide a physiological explanation of why ventilation is greater under hypoxia compared to normoxia.

Unit Four Laboratories

Name: _____

Cardiac Rehabilitation Assessment Laboratory

INTRODUCTION

Maximal exercise testing is used to assess maximal aerobic capacity but is limited in individuals where maximal exercise is contraindicated. Maximal exercise testing is also limited in people whose performance may be limited because of pain or fatigue rather than exertion.

There are several modalities available for the objective evaluation of functional exercise capacity of a diseased population. According to the American Thoracic Society, the most popular clinical exercise tests are stair-climbing, a 6-minute walk test, a shuttle walk test, a cardiac stress test, and a cardiopulmonary exercise test. The goal of clinical exercise testing should be to produce a sufficient level of exercise without physiologic strain.

The goal of exercise testing should be to produce a sufficient level of stress without physiologic or biomechanical strain.

6-MINUTE WALK TEST (6MWT)

The 6MWT is a practical test that requires a 100 ft walk way. Participants should choose their own intensity of exercise and are allowed to stop and rest during the test. Since most ADLs are performed at submaximal levels, the 6MWT may better reflect the functional exercise level for daily physical activities.

Test Procedure:

1. A warm-up period before the test should not be performed. The participant should sit at rest in a chair located near the starting position before the test starts.

2. Measure and record baseline HR and oxygen saturation.

3. Have the participant stand and rate their overall fatigue using the Borg scale.

4. Participant will walk 100 ft and pivot around cone and walk 100 ft back. This counts as one lap. The participant will continue to do this for the entire 6 minutes.

5. The participant will set their own walking pace and is allowed to stop and take breaks during the 6 minutes.

6. After the test record the total number of laps and again ask where they stand for fatigue by the Borg Scale.

7. Measure HR and oxygen saturation.

Unit Four Laboratories   429

TREADMILL TESTS

Treadmill test protocol should progress from low workloads to higher work loads until a predetermined end point is reached. If signs or symptoms develop during the exercise test, then the test should be stopped immediately. Test administrators need to keep in mind protocols that are too long or too short may not truly reflect the participant's functional capacity.

Bruce protocol is better suited for screening younger and/or physically active individuals, while the modified Bruce is used for sedentary individuals. The Naughton protocol is often used in post-MI exercise testing to classify patient into high-risk and low-risk categories.

Bruce Protocol

Bruce	
Mph	%Grade
1.7	10
2.5	12
3.4	14
4.2	16
5.0	18
5.5	20

Modified Bruce	
Mph	%Grade
1.0	0
1.3	5
1.7	10
2.1	10
2.3	11
2.5	12
2.8	12
3.1	13

Naughton Protocol

Mph	%Grade
1.0	0
1.5	0
2.0	3.5
3.0	3.0
3.0	7.0
3.0	10.5
3.0	14
3.0	17.5
3.0	20
3.0	22.5
3.0	25

Participant Sheet

6MWT:

Name: _____

Height:_____ Weight: _____ Age: _____

Number of laps completed _____

HR at rest _____ HR after 6MWT _____

RPE at rest _____ RPE after 6MWT_____

BP at rest_____ BP after 6MWT_____

MODIFIED BRUCE PROTOCOL

Name:_____

Height:_____ Weight: _____ Age: _____

HR at rest _____ BP at rest_____ RPE at rest_____

Post HR_____ Post BP _____ Post RPE _____

Time	Heart rate	RPE

NAUGHTON PROTOCOL

Name: _____

Height:_____   Weight: _____   Age:_____

HR at rest _____   BP at rest_____   RPE at rest_____

Post HR_____   Post BP _____   Post RPE _____

Time	Heart rate	RPE

Questions

1. What is chronic hypertension and what damage is caused by chronic hypertension within the body.

2. The precise mechanism for how regular exercise lowers blood pressure is mainly unknown but what are some significant contributing factors?

3. What is the pathogenesis that CHD follows?

4. What are the reasons for stress testing and explain each one.

5. Explain what the four possible GXT outcomes are.

6. What should a proper exercise prescription do?

Cardiopulmonary Exercise Testing (CPET) Laboratory:

INTERPRETATION OF ECG AND GAS COLLECTION VARIABLES

Objective of this lab: To conduct cardiopulmonary exercise testing and evaluate the ECG and open-circuit spirometry responses in healthy populations as well as in individuals with COPD.

Key Concepts:

1. Ability to set up and prepare an individual for CPET (hook up and administer 12-lead ECG using metabolic systems such as the ParvoMedics to administer the appropriate CPET modality and device protocol).

2. Ability to generate summary and 9 panel reports following completion of CPET.

3. Interpret and explain breath-by-breath changes at rest and during exercise for FeO_2, $FeCO_2$, VO_2, VCO_2, RER, Ve, Vt, RR, breathing reserve (BR), Ve/VO_2, Ve/VCO_2, HR, VO_2–workload relationship, HR–VO_2 relationship, HRR, and O_2 pulse in healthy individuals, those individuals with various types of CVD, and those individuals with various pulmonary diseases.

4. Ability to follow established algorithms for differential diagnosis of various cardiovascular and pulmonary diseases.

5. Ability to identify the ventilatory threshold using the intercept of S1 and S2 of the V-slope graph.

6. Ability to verify the ventilatory threshold using the ventilatory equivalents, Ve/VO_2 and Ve/VCO_2.

7. Ability to identify the suspected period of isocapnic buffering and respiratory compensation using the ventilatory equivalents.

INSTRUCTIONS

1. Have test subject complete a physical activity readiness questionnaire (PAR-Q) and review the responses with your laboratory instructor.

2. With assistance from your instructor perform a FEV1 assessment on the test subject.

3. Calculate predicted MVV using equation MVV = FEV1 × 40 =

_____

4. Perform a modified 12-lead ECG hook up so that the limb leads are moved from the distal limbs to the thorax.

   a. Be certain to practice the skills necessary during ECG hook up to minimize ECG noise/artifact during exercise as well as safety to ensure participant safety while walking/cycling.

5. With assistance from your instructor calibrate the breath-by-breath metabolic system according to manufacturer instructions.

6. Fit the face mask and head gear of the metabolic system onto the subject.

7. Enter test subject's data into the metabolic system and choose maximal treadmill test as the type of test.

8. Select and perform the Bruce protocol in both the metabolic and ECG software.

9. Record rating of perceived exertion at the end of each stage.

10. Encourage participant to continue to push themselves to volitional fatigue.

11. The test should be terminated when the subject requests to stop, fails to conform to the exercise protocol, develops adverse signs and/or symptoms, or experiences any emergency situation.

12. When the test is terminated, immediately begin the active recovery by clicking on the cool down button and allow subject to continue walking at 0% elevation and 1.5 mph. At the same time, have a test technician immediately remove the face mask once the cool down phase is initiated.

13. Upon completion of test, print off the ventilatory threshold graph, the summary report, the 9-panel report, and the text report from the reports tab.

14. Repeat FEV1 test using modified breathing valve that mimics acute COPD.

15. Calculate predicted MVV for modified breathing valve test using equation MVV = FEV1 × 40 = _____

16. Repeat maximal exercise test using modified breathing valve.

Questions

1. List the four most commonly utilized criteria to determine whether a true physiological maximal effort was obtained. For each of these criteria, be certain to list the values obtained from your two CPET and indicate whether the individual values reached criteria for maximal effort for both tests.

2. From panel 2 in the 9-panel report, describe the relationship between HR and time for both CPET. Remember the Bruce protocol is a 3-minute staged protocol with equal (3 METS) increases in workload from one stage to the next and therefore this relationship can be generalized to HR–workload relationship. Is the HR–time (workload) relationship what we expect to see in healthy individuals? Describe how and why this HR–workload relationship may be altered in individuals with left-sided heart failure, chronotropic incompetence, COPD, or obesity.

3. Also in panel 2, describe the O_2 pulse response during both CPET and explain why this measure is often considered the poor man's measure of stroke volume. Be sure to include in your answer the Fick equation and how O_2 pulse is derived from this equation.

Unit Four Laboratories   437

4. Explain how the O_2 pulse in panel 2 might respond to increasing workload in individuals with congestive heart failure as a result of a previous MI. Be sure to include a discussion of the O_2 pulse at rest, with increasing workload, during recovery from exercise in this individual.

5. Calculate the HRR for your test subject during both CPET by subtracting the maximal HR obtained during the CPET from their Age Predicted MaxHR. Discuss whether the HRR might be smaller or larger in individuals with pulmonary disease and potential explanations as to why the HRR is altered in this population.

6. Looking at panel 5 of the 9 panel, describe the HR–Vo_2 relationship for both CPET. Discuss how this relationship may be altered in pulmonary diseases and in cardiovascular diseases. What other condition might affect the HR–Vo_2 relationship.

7. From panel 1 of the 9 panel, discuss the relationship between ventilation (VE) and time (workload) for both CPET. If there are different slopes to this relationship, be sure to discuss why the VE/workload slope is different even though workload increments are equal in progression. Confirm with panel 7 as well as your text report what the maximum VE is for your test.

438   Unit Four Laboratories

8. Determine your test subjects breathing reserve for both CPET at maximal intensity by subtracting the maximal VE from question number 7 from the calculated MVV at the beginning of this lab. Discuss what the breathing reserve may look like for individuals with CVD or pulmonary disease.

9. From panel 7 of your 9 panel, explain the relationship observed between Vt (l) and VE (l/min) for both CPET. How might this relationship be altered in individuals with restrictive lung diseases and in individuals with obstructive pulmonary disease?

10. Reviewing your responses from the previous questions, what physio logical systems may be limiting maximal performance? Discuss which physiological systems may not be limiting in maximal performance.

Unit Four Laboratories   439